Lotus Lake, Dragon Pool

FURTHER ENCOUNTERS IN YOGA AND ZEN

by

Trevor Leggett

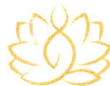

Trevor Leggett Adhyatma Yoga Trust

Published by Trevor Leggett Adhyatma Yoga Trust
PO Box 362
KINGS LYNN
PE31 8WQ
United Kingdom
www.tlayt.org

First published by Charles E Tuttle Company, Inc in 1994

Printed in the United Kingdom

ISBN (Paperback edition): 978-1-911467-02-1
ISBN (Ebook edition): 978-1-911467-03-8

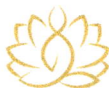

Trevor Leggett Adhyatma Yoga Trust

To the late Hari Prasad Shastri
in whose life and words
the ancient traditions drew new breath
these translations and transcriptions
are reverently dedicated

Table of Contents

Publisher's Foreword

TREVOR LEGGETT collected many teaching stories from the Indian Yoga tradition and from the Chinese and Japanese Zen traditions drawn from various sources both ancient and modern: for example they may be from an old temple magazine, folk stories, from the oral tradition or sometimes from his own experience. These stories can provide inspiration to beginners as well as those with some knowledge and experience of Yoga and Zen. Their function is to strike a spark and if they do so they should be pondered daily for some weeks to find the deeper points. The author explains this in more detail in the introduction to the companion volume to this book, 'Encounters in Yoga and Zen - Meetings of Cloth and Stone' which can be found on the Trust website tlayt.org at Audio tracks - Going Further into a Story.

THE PICTURES in this book were brushed by Jacques Allais and generously given to Trevor Leggett for this book. The pictures are in the Suiboku style in which Jacques Allais was an expert. The style gives a hint for the focusing of meditation practice, providing the perfect complement to Trevor Leggett's text.

Lotus Lake

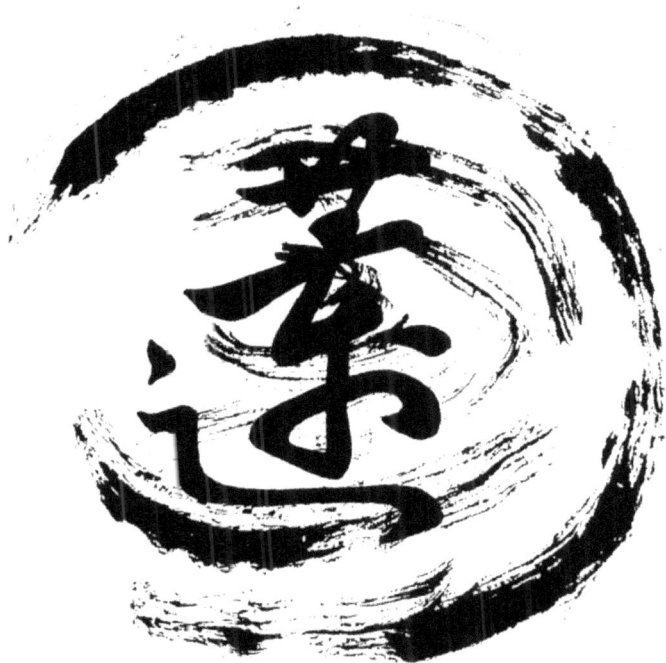

The Magistrate

A TEACHER of the Yoga of the Bhagavad-Gita came to the district and set up a school in a village there. When this was reported to the local magistrate (the chief administrative officer for the district), he was displeased. He was a follower of a Western philosopher who held that traditional religion and its compulsive morality was the cause of many of the ills of man.

The magistrate had a great love for the people of the district, and worked night and day to bring them to what he saw as modern and progressive views. He therefore put many obstacles in the way of the yoga teacher, and for a time was successful in turning public opinion against him.

When he heard that the school was also teaching secular subjects to the local children (admittedly poorly served by the present arrangements, because of the poverty of the district), he briefed the school inspector to apply the most stringent tests to the teaching methods. The latter, however, reported favourably, and in fact two of the yoga teacher's disciples had been school-teachers and were teaching very ably for a tiny salary. In five years, three of the pupils of this school obtained state scholarships to go on to a high school in the capital, and then to the university. Such a thing had never happened before.

The magistrate's attitude began to soften. Though he never even came to meet the yoga master, he used his influence to help him in various ways, and indirectly conveyed to the group that if they were in difficulties, they could approach him through a designated intermediary. The disciples concluded that though

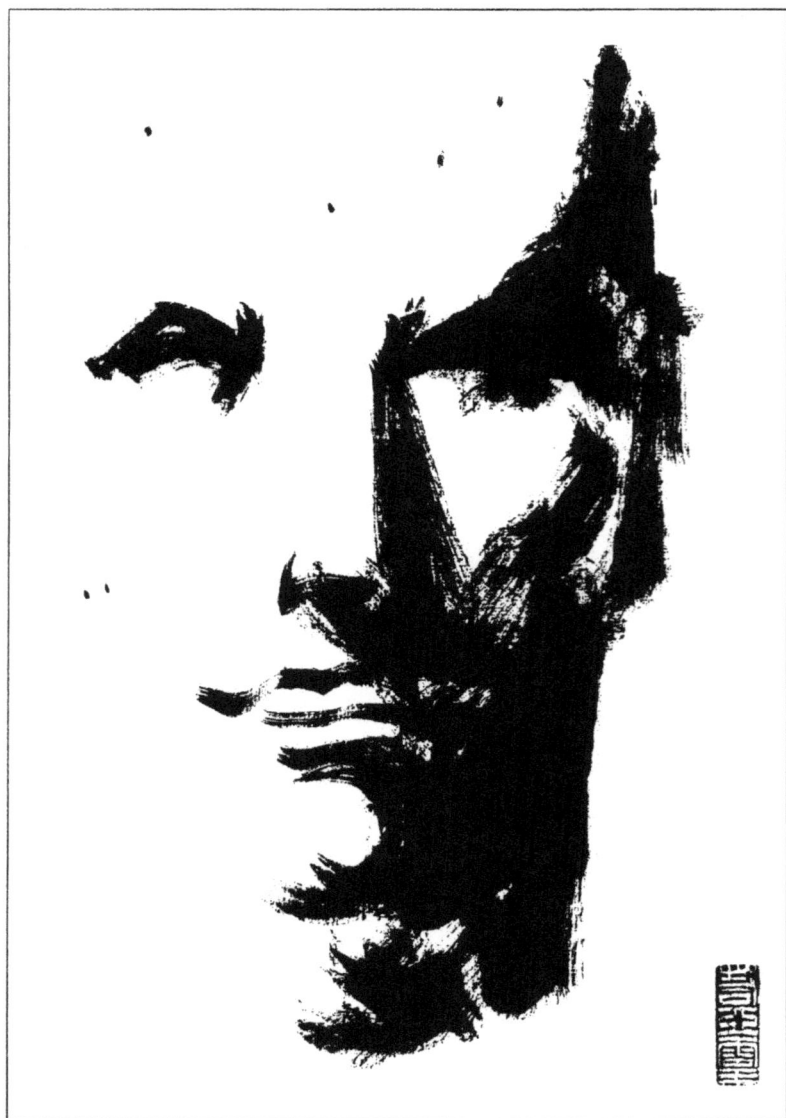

the magistrate could hardly reverse his previous stance, he had in fact become a religious devotee in private.

After some years he fell ill. He went to the capital for a major operation, but returned little better, and it was generally assumed that he had come home to die. The teacher sent a disciple, with no instructions except to present himself. He was refused admission. He sat down on the ground in an inconspicuous place not far from the door. As night came on, his body shivered in the cold, and a servant who saw him brought a mat and a straw coat; he then reported to his master that the disciple was still waiting.

Late in the night, the master asked, "Is he still there?"

"Yes," was the answer. "I gave him some food."

"Well, let him in," ordered the sick man. "I have decided to see him."

As the disciple bowed on the threshold, the magistrate said irritably, "You've come to preach to me, I suppose."

"I won't say a word unless you tell me to," promised the brahmachari.

"Well, I have decided that I may as well tell you—in fact, I must tell you in fairness—that I have never believed that superstitious stuff you are propagating among the people. And I don't believe it now. But I have seen that your teacher could get people to cooperate, and to work and study, on the basis of pleasing God; and I had found that they just couldn't see clearly enough when I explained to them the same things, on the basis of enlightened self-interest. And I concluded that perhaps the religious phase is a necessary one, to get them moving. Afterwards, as they become better informed, they will discard it. So I gave some help to your efforts; the dogmas do seem to be of some immediate benefit to the people, and ultimately they are bound to destroy themselves.

"Now I've told you. I felt suddenly that your master was entitled to know, to prevent any misunderstandings later. I hope it isn't too much of a shock to you. I don't suppose you have any text to cover this case, have you?"

"My Lord, we have," the disciple told him. "It is in the Gita, where the Lord says that in whatever form people worship Him, that same faith He makes unwavering."

There was a long silence.

The magistrate said feebly, "Is there any other text that comes to your mind?"

The brahmachari replied softly, "Yes—He sees, who sees the Lord standing in all beings, the undying in the dying."

Another silence.

"Anything else?" The magistrate's voice was very weak.

The brahmachari came and knelt by the bed with his palms joined. "O my Lord, you cannot tease me any more. I see you clearly now."

A great surprise came over the magistrate's face; and then he died.

The brahmachari called the servant, and told him, "Your master is gone now, and well gone." The servant stood in the doorway looking toward the dead man for a little. Then he said in a choked voice, "He was a great man. Yes, and he was a good man too. They said he was strict and hard. Well, he was; he was strict and hard. I should know that; I served him for twelve years. But it was for our own good, and I know that too. And he was much stricter with himself, and much harder on himself. He was so anxious that he shouldn't leave anything undone, so anxious. I don't think I ever saw him smile, he was so anxious."

He took a step toward the bed, and peered toward the face.

"But tell me—I'm not seeing very well just now—that's a smile there, isn't it?" He caught the brahmachari's arm. "It's true, isn't it? He's smiling now, isn't he?"

"Yes," the brahmachari told him. "He's smiling now."

Do Good

"NOT MUCH thanks in this world when you do a kindly action," grumbled a disciple. "They at once try to find something wrong with it, and if they can't find something wrong with it, they find something wrong with you. Seems to make them feel better somehow."

"I heard a good saying in one of the devotional schools," remarked a senior. "Apparently their teacher used to say: 'Do good, and be abused.' But he told them that the resistance and abuse against good deeds was like the bow-wave when a ship is moving forward strongly; in a way it is a confirmation, and should not be resented too much."

"Yes, I know, I know. It's all very clever and elevating, but the fact is that when spiteful things are actually being said, when a well-meant action is deliberately twisted to seem self-seeking—it's a bit different then. I haven't got the patience to listen to all that venomous stuff."

"We have the saying in our own school: Do Good and Go. They tell us not to hang about, either for praise or blame."

"Still, one's bound to hear something even as one goes … and one remark can be as wounding as twenty."

"Well, I suppose in your case we'll have to amend the saying. Try this then: Do Good and Run!"

Self-Examination

TWO FRIENDS who belonged to a group practising interior training were given the practice of self-examination. "At the end of the day, sit down for a few minutes and try to see where you have gone wrong: make attempts to correct the faults." One of them, a desperately conscientious man, raised the point when they next had a meeting with the teacher.

"I find myself overwhelmed when I do self-examination," he said. "I feel absolutely crushed. It seems to have been all blunders and meanness and weakness. I can't get rid of the thought of them afterwards, either. Sometimes I can't sleep."

The teacher said, "There is another way for people like you. You need not do formal self-examination. Whenever you think of your mistakes, turn your mind on to the Lord. Create vividly in your mind the scenes from the life of His incarnations. This will free you. Make friends with the lion, and you will not be bothered by jackals." Then he turned to the other, and asked him how he found the practice.

"Oh, I don't have trouble at all," he replied. "I've come to realize that humility is the secret of self-examination. If the thought comes up that I have failed in virtue, I just think, the Lord did not give me the strength. If the idea comes that I have not prayed, I think, He did not give me a devotional nature. If it occurs to me that I have not studied the holy scriptures, to find out how to approach Him, then I say, after all, He did not give me the head for that. When I realize that I have not been very helpful to my fellow men, I think, He did not bless me with loving kindness.

"All I am and all I do and all I think—it is all from Him. What have I to repent of, what have I to correct? It is all His, nothing of mine at all."

"There might be just one thing of your own in all this," said the teacher.

"And what is that?"

"Perhaps ... a tiny bit of pride in your own cleverness?"

Last Words

A TEACHER of the Gita Yoga had as a disciple an Englishman brought up to restrain expression of feeling. The teacher approved of this as a basis, but got him to take part in amateur theatricals and public speaking so that there should be some creative expression. The Englishman's mother was sceptical (though she had been baptized) and often sarcastic about religion. They lived far apart, and when they did meet he never talked about his beliefs and practice. She had a vague idea that he was inclined to some strange Oriental cult, but she would dismiss the subject of religion in a few sharp words if ever it appeared on the conversational horizon. She recognized that he was a good son to her. When finally she fell very ill, he took her into his home to look after in the final stages.

Now the teacher had told this disciple, as he told all of them, not to feel he was giving up the religion into which he had been born. He recommended him to read from the New Testament every day, which he did with slowly increasing interest. Later he took to having a crucifix by his bed during the night.

One day the teacher asked about the mother, and hearing that she was very weak, said, "The Gita declares that the last thought of the dying person may be very important. If when you are there you become aware that your mother is about to die, say into her ear, 'Jesus loves you.'"

The disciple gulped. Suppose, he thought to himself, Mother didn't die but recovered for a bit; he could imagine her reaction. Only the week before, a well-meaning friend had sent her a postcard with angels pictured on it, and the inscription below, "When we pass over, they are waiting to greet us on the other side." His mother had snorted contemptuously, and remarking, "How do they know, I wonder?" told him to throw it in the wastepaper basket.

Then he pondered that after all he had only been told to do it if he knew definitely that she was dying, and he could never be completely certain of that. On the other hand, this had been an instruction from the teacher, so there must be circumstances in which it would apply. His mind wavered to and fro for a long while but in the end he made up his mind to do it.

When the time came, however, and his mother lay dying before him, he found himself so embarrassed that he could not bring the words out. He stood silently and prayed. Afterwards, telling the whole story to another pupil, a close friend, he ended, "I just couldn't do it. I often worry about it now; I feel it was a big failure, but I just couldn't do it. I couldn't let Mother go over with her last thought not 'Jesus loves you,' but 'Jimmy's gone barmy!' Because that's what she would have thought."

Some years later, the Englishman himself died, alone and in the night. He was lying peacefully and there had been no struggle, but it seemed that he had woken before it happened, as he was found holding the crucifix. His friend one day discussed with a senior the story as he knew it, and remarked, "I think our teacher must have made a little miscalculation there, when he told him to say those words 'Jesus loves you' to his mother. After all, he must have known Jimmy wouldn't be able to say them: it was absolutely impossible for someone brought up like him. And it worried him a lot; he often thought how he had failed."

The senior, a woman, laughed at the story, but added, "Not absolutely impossible, you know. If it had been absolutely impossible, he wouldn't have worried about it. The Gita says that the Lord is in the heart of every being, so nothing's absolutely impossible, is it? I agree that our teacher knew it was highly unlikely that he would get over the obstacles and say these words. But the point is, he thought about it often. No doubt there was a feeling of worry, of having failed, but still, he was thinking about it.

"And when he himself woke up in the night and realized that he was dying, and just had the strength to reach for that crucifix, what do you suppose came to his mind? It was those words. He'd failed to say them before, but they didn't fail him then."

Anger

IN THE sermon it was remarked in passing that in the Eastern traditions it was generally held that the worst sin was anger leading to injury to others, whereas in Christianity it seemed that sexual license was worse; in English, for instance, the very word *immorality* had overtones of sexual transgressions.

This part of the sermon was reported to a Christian who lived in the neighbourhood, and he later tackled the preacher on the point, adding, "I get angry myself, but only with good reason, so I don't regard it as particularly sinful. After all, when Christ drove the money-changers from the Temple, he showed anger, and he was unquestionably right. When I get angry, it's the same thing."

The preacher took him outside onto the grass and gave him a big stone. He told him, "Throw this stone on the ground with all your force." He flung it down and it made a great dent in the ground. The priest removed the stone and said, "Come back when that mark has gone." It took some weeks before the mark was gradually obliterated by the rains and by people walking over it.

Then the priest said, "This is like your anger. Now take up the stone again." They went to a still lake and the Christian was asked to throw the stone as hard as he could into the water. It made a tremendous splash, and the ripples went to the edge of the lake. But in five minutes all was completely calm again. The preacher continued, "And that is the anger of a Christ. It is just a passing thing, just for this event, and it doesn't do any

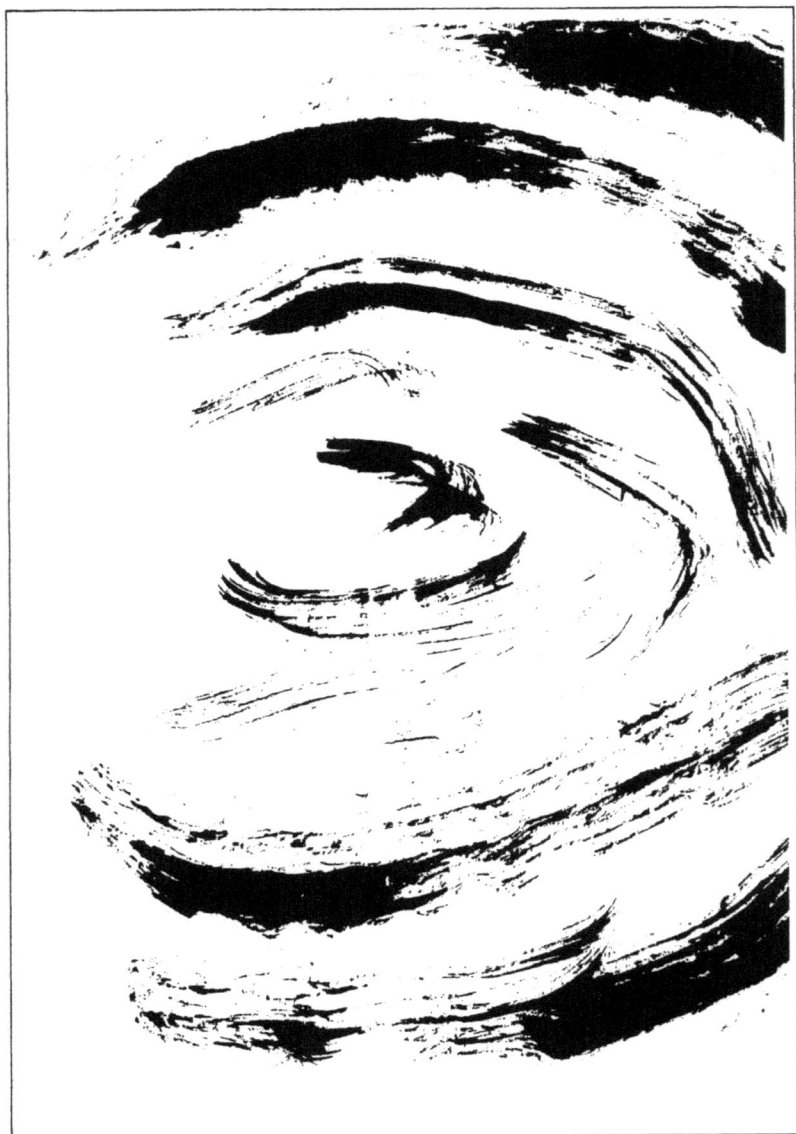

damage. When you struck the ground with your stone, some little insects were killed; but all you have just done here was to disturb the water momentarily, and it was even good for the plants at the edge of the water."

The Christian was impressed, but did not want to give in so easily, and argued, "You've told me that my anger remains, and has lasting effects, whereas His anger is momentary and bears no malice. But still, at the moment of anger, mine is the same as the anger of Christ, isn't it?"

The priest said, "It may seem so, but it is not really so. Take the example of water again. Suppose a smoothly flowing stream, and suddenly it is dammed by a landslide or something like that. It piles up before the obstacle; it froths and swirls as if in frustration. It looks angry, so to say. But then, it goes round, and soon creates a new channel round the obstacle, and is flowing smoothly as before. There is no permanent mark, and there is no fixed attitude, no posture."

Habits

"I DON'T see why we are asked to come to meditation and devotion practice classes. Surely the whole point of yoga is to develop the consciousness in the ordinary affairs of life, so we ought to practise them in that field. If we don't do that, they are basically useless for life." This sort of objection is very common, especially among ambitious or property-loving disciples. A teacher once answered in this way:

"If you practise only in the ordinary life, your practice will be affected by the associations of that life. You may be unconscious of the distortion, but it will still be there. It used to be said among forgers of signatures that it is relatively easy to make a near imitation of someone else's signature. The really difficult thing is to prevent some of one's own characteristic letter-formations from subtly influencing the movement of the pen. To rule this out, skillful forgers used to practise a signature upside down, purely as a pattern. That ruled out any traces of the forger's own handwriting. There were no familiar associations to activate them.

"In the same way, in ordinary life you may try to imitate the conduct of a yogin, but the associations will subtly affect your behaviour. You will find that very often your good intentions lead to poor results. Without some inner inspiration, you will find yourself backing wrong horses, so to say.

"By practising regularly in circumstances free from familiar associations, you can build up clear inner awareness. Then your actions will be in accordance with the inner current of things. Of course, before this happens, we have to do our best on the basis of traditional right and wrong, but we must not expect too much from what we do. The most important thing is to practise to attain some inner calm; it is in calm that we can act well. At the beginning, that practice has to be done in special circumstances. Later, it can be maintained in rough waters as well as smooth."

Honour

A GREAT scholar, a devout man, was suddenly offered a very high position in the political field. It would be largely prestige, but he thought that he would be able to do a good deal to encourage and support scholarship and religion from that eminence. He would, however, have to spend a good bit of his time in official ceremonial, and to that extent his own work would suffer.

After some hesitation, he accepted the honour and duly received many telegrams of congratulation, and also a large number of small presents in accordance with the custom of the country.

A friend of his, a spiritual teacher, sent him a little packet. When he opened it, he found that it contained chocolates wrapped up in gold paper to look like coins.

Prayers Answered

BEFORE ONE enters a yogic path, it is natural to pray to the Lord for legitimate accessories to a natural life, with a view to share them also with others. The prayers are answered, unless they would be fatal to that person's spiritual growth. When he has entered on a path, however, the yogin is expected to rely on his own Great Self, and not to pray for anything at all, either for himself or others.

An idealistic schoolmaster in a small village complained to his teacher that if only he had a larger place, he could do much more for the children of the neighbourhood. "Surely I may pray for that?" he said. "I do not understand our rule which forbids praying for things. Surely it cannot be wrong to pray for that?"

"Devote yourself to realization of your self in God," said the teacher, "and you will do much more good, to the children as well, than any actions in a new schoolplace."

"But in the meantime," persisted the schoolmaster, "surely, surely ..."

"Well," said the teacher finally, "there is one kind of prayer which is allowed. It is nearly always answered rather quickly. But it is rather difficult to do, and ..."

"Tell me, tell me," broke in the other.

"Here it is then. The prayer must be uttered, but you must not be conscious that it is uttered. And it must be uttered with a mouth by which you have never sinned."

The schoolmaster listened to this, and took his leave in some bewilderment. Some time later he told the teacher that he found the prayer quite impossible. "How can I utter it and be unconscious of it? And anyway, I am ruled out because I have sometimes misused my tongue shamefully, as I now realize. I thought at first it was a bit cruel to tell me such impossible things, but of course I did persist in asking. Well, I have put the idea aside, and gone back to my yoga practices. As a matter of fact, it has been a sort of stimulus to them, I don't know why."

Some months later, the local mayor told the schoolmaster that the inspectors had reported very favourably on his work, and that he himself had organized a petition to the Education Ministry. There was a new minister who seized the chance to show a human face (and get publicity) by agreeing to build a larger school in the remote village.

The schoolmaster took the wonderful news to his teacher, who said, "Let us bow together to thank God for answering your prayer."

"But I didn't make the prayer. You said it had to be uttered without my being conscious of it, and by a mouth with which I had never sinned. That wasn't possible, and it wasn't done."

"It was possible, and it was done," the teacher told him. "The prayer was uttered by others, by the parents of the children you have helped. You weren't conscious of it. Then it was uttered by their mouths, and you have never sinned with their mouths.

"Worship of God through the bodies and minds of others, influenced unknown to you by your yogic life and meditation, is worship of the purest kind: it cannot be polluted even by a temporary association with things."

Proclaimed Wisdom

A KING heard about a special thirty days' discipline by which he could be blessed with the gift of Proclaimed Wisdom— namely wisdom and the ability to declare it. The discipline was harsh, but the king was delighted to discover that it contained no requirement as to mental control, which would have ruled him out. The only necessity was endurance. He managed to follow the drastic reduction in his diet, the total abstinence from alcohol and opium, the limitation of sleep to three hours, but he found it increasingly difficult to keep himself away from his queen and concubines. On the twenty-seventh day he realized that he was not going to be able to do so by his will alone.

He had himself dressed in poor clothes, and then the chief minister locked him in a deep dungeon underneath the palace. A stupid and fanatical pair of guards were borrowed from the train of a visiting ambassador, who told them (as he had been told) that a dangerous conspirator was to be kept in that dungeon, and that they were being given the privilege of guarding him for the three days. They were only to pass him in some poor food and water. They could not speak the language, of course, but they were also to pay no attention to signs.

For three days and nights the king shouted and raved and pleaded and wept, and fell ill and nearly died, and cursed the guards for their stupidity. They followed their instructions. On the completion of the last three days, the guards were returned with a reward, and the king (an exhausted shadow of himself, but in the royal robes) waited in the courtyard.

Soon after dawn a heavenly messenger came flying toward the kingdom, bearing a little pot which contained dew that had fallen on a certain altar on a certain sacred mountain, collected every morning. When drunk, it would give the blessing of Proclaimed Wisdom. As he neared the capital, the messenger saw some girls bathing in a stream, and found himself suddenly submerged by a tidal wave of desire. He put the pot on a rock at the top of a high cliff, and went down to them. When he came back he found the pot upset and the nectar all spilt; a squirrel had investigated it, knocked it over, and fled.

The messenger, aghast, refilled the pot with water from the stream, and went on. He alighted in the courtyard and presented the pot to the king, who in the presence of all the people, slowly drank it. The audience prostrated themselves.

Under the pretense of giving an initiation, the messenger drew near the king and whispered what had happened, continuing, "It will take a month till the pot can be filled again. When it is, I shall bring it to you secretly. It will be my last commission, as I shall have to pass three lives as a quadruped, having become a quadruped on my way here. You will be expected to proclaim wisdom. My own wisdom is limited, but I can tell you some things which you can say to gain time till you actually drink the water and can speak wisdom from yourself. For instance, I can tell you the method of controlling passion."

"You are hardly the one to do that," retorted the king. "But in any case, that's not the sort of thing I want. Tell me some things that are going to happen, so that I can prophesy to my people."

"O king," said the heavenly messenger, "it was the great wave of your frustrated desire which overwhelmed me on the way to your palace; I had never expected to meet anything like that outside hell. It took me by surprise. I do know the method of controlling passion, but I did not apply it, and I shall suffer for that failure. As to prophecies, I can tell you only one

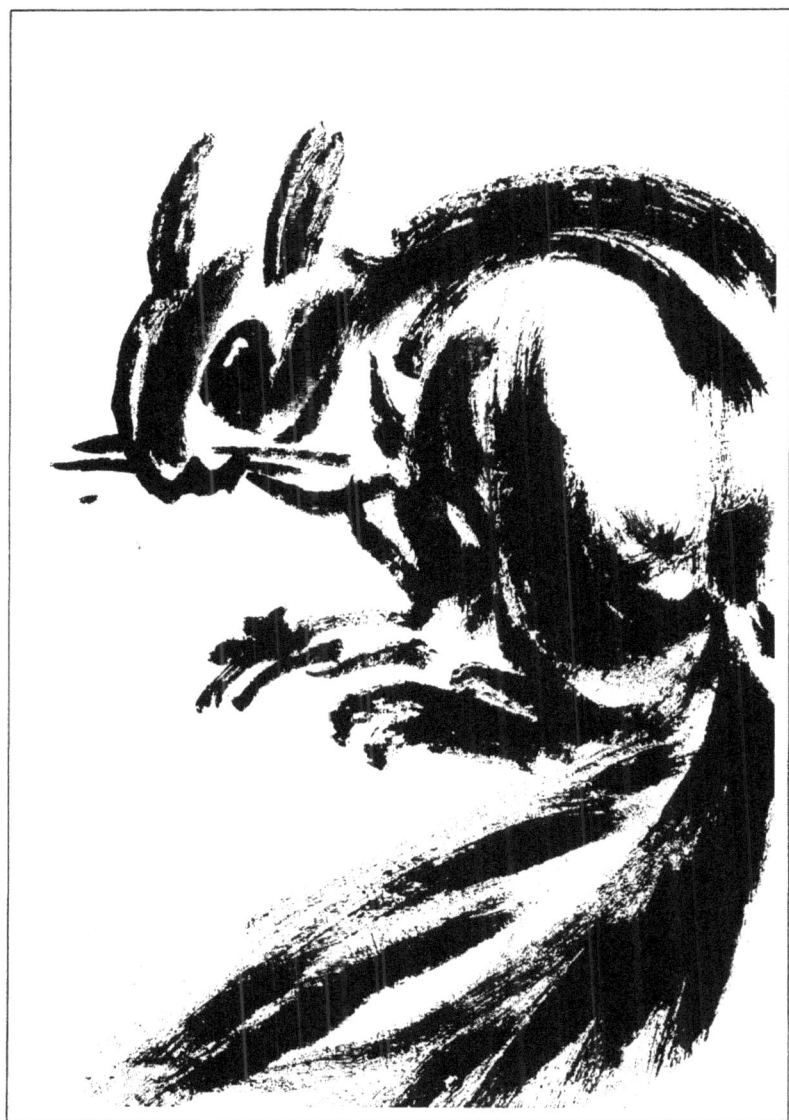

thing: There is bound to be an earthquake tonight, as a result of the thwarting of the proper course of things. After that, you must bluff your way with ambiguous announcements, as most oracles do. Don't answer more than one question a day."

He took his leave and rose into the air. The people raised their heads and the king motioned them to get up. "O my people," he shouted, "do not remain in your houses tonight. Sleep in the streets or in the fields. There is going to be an earthquake!"

The people hurried home and brought out their furniture and beds into the streets, while the king had everything and everyone taken from the palace. Sure enough, there was something of an earthquake which brought some houses down. But thanks to the king's warning, no one was injured except a few who had refused to believe.

Next day in the court, the king announced that for the next month he would answer just one question each morning. A minister asked, "In the neighbouring state, a general is rebelling against the king (a different one). Will he be successful or not?" The king did not like the neighbouring monarch, and on an impulse said, "The general will be successful." That king, who had heard about the earthquake prediction and the events that led up to it, at once made his submission to the general in order to save needless bloodshed in a lost cause.

Next day the king was asked about a famous poet and writer who had become ill. The king did not like this man either, and said, "The illness will be fatal." When this was reported to the writer he turned pale, lost all desire to eat, and died.

In this way the king created the future by his predictions, which became more and more potent as each one was confirmed.

After a month, the heavenly messenger appeared secretly in the king's bedroom, with a pot full of the nectar. "This," he said, "will give you true wisdom, not these prophecies you have been making, which have nothing to do with wisdom. When you are wise, you will not make them."

"Then you can keep your nectar," snapped back the king. "I am satisfied that what I am doing is far better than preaching to people about controlling passions and that sort of thing. What I do has real results." (Soon afterwards he had his first and only failure, having predicted that he himself would live forever.)

The messenger took the pot, and rose into the air, not knowing what to do. With his divine sight he saw another messenger, on his way to give spiritual illumination to a saintly man. He said, "I will come along with you, and give him what I have as well."

"But he does not speak at all," said the other. "He has taken a vow of silence because the people round here are such terrible gossips. He may have the wisdom, but I do not see how he will be able to proclaim it."

Nevertheless the blessing of Proclaimed Wisdom was given along with the blessing of Illumination. They slipped the two potions into the drink of herbs which one of the saint's disciples prepared for him each evening. When the saint tasted the sweetness of it, he looked inquiringly at the disciple, who stared back blankly. The master drank it up without pursuing the point; he supposed that the disciple had put in something sugary without realizing how sweet it was.

Thereafter, when the people of the town saw the saint, they often found a sort of peace coming into them; their passions were quieted, and they had courage and inspiration to face the battles of life.

One man, who was shouldering heavy responsibilities, had always been a target for jealous gossip and envious slanders, along with the host of anxieties and worries connected with his position. He saw the saint, on his way to visit a dying woman, passing through the monsoon rain. He was not huddling under the eaves like others on the street, but walking calmly through the wall of water, head thrown back and obviously enjoying the feel of the warm rain, not at all put out by the soaking of his simple dress. It made a vivid picture, which remained in the mind of the onlooker. Later on, when that worried man was confronted with the usual mosquito swarm of his anxieties, the image of the holy figure in the rain came to him, rising before his inner eye again and again. At first obscurely and later more clearly, he found that in himself there was something which could walk serenely through the downpour of inner apprehensions and outer disparagement. He felt that it was all nothing more than a monsoon rain, which would pass away of itself.

Another man of the town had undertaken, or rather been burdened with, a long task which seemed never-ending. He felt he would never be free from it. Sometimes he would work energetically for a week or so, but it seemed to make no impression on the magnitude of what remained, and then he would sink into apathy. Whether he tried hard or did nothing, it made no appreciable difference.

The town was not far from a desert, and if a strong wind blew up from a certain direction, the houses on that side would have their little gardens covered with sand drifts. One of these was the saint's small place. The townsman happened to pass that way after a sandstorm, and he saw that the garden was piled with sand, round the flowers and bushes, on their leaves, everywhere. He saw the holy man with a tiny brush, slowly and rhythmically sweeping sand off the leaves into a little pan, and thought to himself, "At that rate, it will take him weeks to get it clear."

He noticed in the neighboring garden a little boy of about three, who was piling up the sand with his hands into little hills and then laughing as they collapsed. Looking at the two, he realized that the saint too was enjoying the shifting patterns made by the sand as he brushed it. He felt a sort of cool breeze in his heart. When he got home, the endlessness of his own task

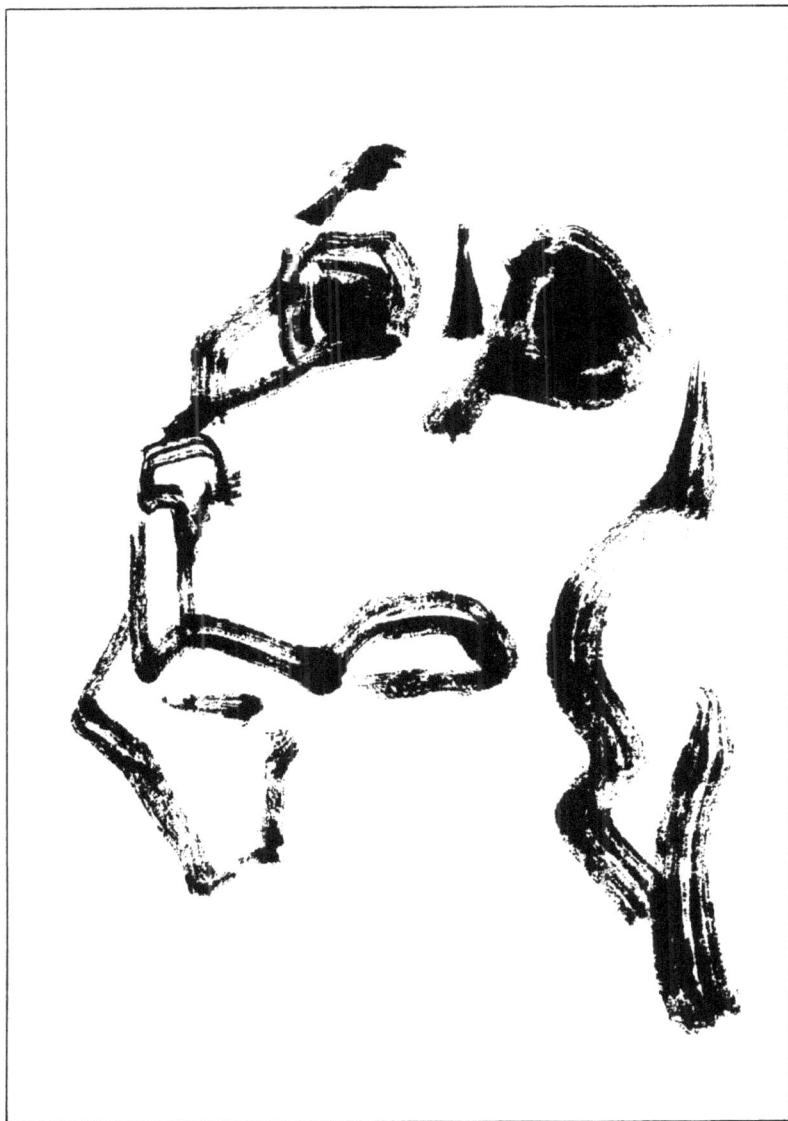

took on a new dimension. He found he could now enjoy each little bit of it as he did it, without thinking further, and felt himself freed from a crushing burden.

In the last years of the saint's life, a stray dog turned up. It looked as if it had traveled a long way, and gone through terrible experiences. It attached itself to him, following him around with great devotion, but never getting in the way. It seemed to understand many things about his life. One day when the dog was sitting on the little verandah beside the teacher, two disciples in the garden below were discussing traditional stories about aspirants who for some fault had to undergo animal existence, but nevertheless retained their memory and higher awareness through the time of imprisonment in a lower body. One of them was saying confidently, "Oh, rather impossible, I'd have thought." He recalled one of the stories about a camel, and said rhetorically, "How could he retain spiritual consciousness during a camel incarnation? The brain of a camel simply couldn't entertain the thoughts." He suddenly felt the dog's intelligent eyes on him, and stopped with an inexplicable sense of embarrassment.

Above, the saint nodded, and patted the dog affectionately.

The Judge

(There is a hint of this story, though not the main point, in Kipling's short "On the Gate." He calls his main human character St. Peter; as this has the necessary associations for most Western readers, it is followed here to save explanations.)

AN ANGEL was appointed to judge one whole generation of humans. He had been given a limited omniscience and omnipresence, so that he could live through their lives with those whom he would afterwards judge.

When the last member of the generation had died, he was told to get ready for his task. But he was instructed to pay his respects to St. Peter first.

In a clear voice, the angel explained to St. Peter, "I shall not judge these humans from the outside. I was given the grace to be with them, in fact in them, every moment of their lives. I have known all the difficulties and temptations they were subject to. I have lived through their agonies of indecision, I have succeeded with them and failed with them. I have given my life to save my friends, and I have betrayed my friends to save my own skin. I have been a compassionate helper, and I have been a murderer."

"How do you propose to judge them?" asked St. Peter.

"I have the record of all that happened, and another, of all that ought to have happened. I shall compare the lists, and judge on that basis. As I said, I know their free will is limited. Though I am an angel and absolutely pure, I have been through it all with them. I shall take everything into consideration, of course. I am fully qualified to be a judge.

St. Peter said, "For that, you still lack one thing."

"And what is that?"

"You are an angel, and absolutely pure. You don't know what it is to need forgiveness yourself."

The angel looked at St. Peter, and St. Peter looked at the angel.

Then the angel whispered, "Yes, I've been self-righteous and arrogant. Forgive me," and he knelt.

St. Peter blessed him and said, "Now go and judge."

Tail, No Tail

A FOREIGNER visiting a Himalayan region for the first time was impressed by the sight of troops of langur monkeys, dropping fearlessly down almost vertical cliff faces by catching on projecting branches of trees. He noticed the use they could make of their prehensile tails, often much longer than their bodies. Some of them would hang by their tails.

He happened to meet an English-speaking yogin, and mentioned it to him. The yogin said, "These monkeys are sacred because of the association with Hanuman, but their physical form itself teaches a lesson. Their name comes from a Sanskrit word meaning 'tailed one,' and it is one of their central attributes. If that tail were strapped to the body, so that the monkey could not free it, it would become atrophied, its owner would feel pain and probably soon die. If the monkey does not use the tail, it will sicken, and finally kill him.

"Man, on the other hand, has no external tail. So not using a tail does him no harm at all; he has not got one. But he has got a higher mind, a buddhi, which is one of his central attributes. If he does not use that, he will suffer. It will spiritually atrophy, sicken, and finally kill his awareness.

"The monkey, in whom the buddhi is as yet asleep and not functioning, does not suffer from not using it. For practical purposes, he has not got one.

"But when in the course of time the monkey has become a man, if he neglects to use the buddhi, he is going against something in himself. The result will be intense suffering, and a temporary check to his further progress.

"There is an ancient epic called Ramayana, which depicts an earlier age when the display of maya was not the same as the present one. The monkey Hanuman is shown at the beginning with his higher intelligence clouded. But after meeting the divine incarnation Rama, he becomes not only wise but a prince of devotees. In the story, however (which has a symbolic meaning for the present day), some of his external behaviour remains primitive. Though he is superior in character to any of the humans, he still can use his tail to great effect in the war against the demon Ravana."

Powers

IN A remote area of an undeveloped country, a river came rushing out from the mountains, dividing just afterwards. Still further on, the two streams joined up again. So there were two huge arcs of flowing water enclosing a long, wide island. The surrounding terrain was mostly desert, but the villages beside the river could live reasonably well. No general irrigation schemes had ever been developed.

Once a small landslide blocked one of the branches of the river just below the division; all the villagers living on that arc of the river cooperated to clear it, thus rescuing their water supply.

The village situated at the spot where the river divided realized that they could dam up one branch of the river by felling trees into it, thus starving the villages on that arc of water. They trained themselves in the use of weapons. When they were an efficient fighting force, they began to blackmail all the villages, threatening to cut off their water supplies, either by blocking one arc alone, or even diverting the whole river into a deep cavern reputed to be bottomless. A few of the villages refused to pay the tribute, and attempted to conquer the village that was demanding it. But they were defeated in battle by the trained armed men and had to capitulate. The armed village now became aristocrats, living on tribute enforced by their arms.

A new, enlightened government came into power, and the head village realized that at some time in the future their monopoly and aristocratic life would be threatened. Looking far ahead, they selected a very bright boy who had a strong sense of village patriotism; they changed his name and falsified the records to make it appear that he had been born in another village. Then they arranged for his higher education at the capital, with special attention to agriculture and planning. They directed him to work his way up in the ministry which would ultimately control the affairs of this area. He was successful, and became one of the young assistants to the Minister.

As they had hoped, he was asked to prepare a plan for this area. It was thought that his local knowledge would be useful. When he presented the plan to the Minister, one of the proposals was to end the monopoly and tribute, and build a dam and reservoir to bring a whole wide area under cultivation.

The Minister scanned the papers and remarked, "You yourself come from that village, do you not? It has been kept secret, of course, but we have some good intelligence agents."

His assistant looked surprised, but admitted, "Yes, it is true. But all that has to go. It is holding up progress."

The Minister nodded, and the plan was published.

When the news reached the village, the father and uncles were horrified, and came in a group to see their protégé. His father burst out, "What are you doing? We arranged for your education, everything, so that you could keep our traditional position safe. And now you are using your power against us. Have you no loyalty, no gratitude?"

"Father!" said the young official. "Why do you suppose that I am entrusted with this power? It is because I can see the interests of the whole country, and not just the interests of our little village. If I were still thinking in terms of the advantage of one village, I should never have this official position. Our people will be given a good pension, but the blackmailing profits will cease. This power has come to me because I have studied and can see clearly the whole area. I cannot now shut my eyes and be aware of only the tiny area of personal interest."

Obedience

"YOUR DISCIPLES treat you with great reverence," remarked a visitor to a teacher. "I suppose they follow literally what you tell them, and you have to be careful. They are always saying, 'The teacher wants this,' or 'The teacher doesn't like that.'"

"They do follow literally what I tell them," replied the teacher, "so long as they agree with it. If they don't agree with it, they interpret it as a joke, or a sort of riddle which they have to interpret. Then they interpret it into what they want, which is sometimes the very reverse of what I have said."

"How could they do that?" marveled the visitor.

"Oh, quite easily," said the teacher. "For instance, I tell them not to swallow the teachings I give without examining them. I ask them to think for themselves; if they have a sensible objection, I tell them to raise it. But some of them think that to do so would show a lack of faith in me. So their doubts never really get resolved; they only get buried.

"Some of them devote themselves to what they call service, but which is really self-display and domination. Good cooks take charge of the kitchen, and make quite unnecessarily elaborate meals for us; they have no time to practise yoga. When I say that the cooking should be done by all in turn, they say, 'Oh, but we couldn't have badly cooked food served to the teacher.' And one of the expert cooks goes into the kitchen just the same and bosses the beginner who is cook that week.

"I tell them not to reverence me, but to practise for God-realization and Self-realization. But they think that is all my holy humility.

"In fact, they do everything I say, if it agrees with their own preconceived ideas. And as the yogic training is based on giving up preconceived ideas, what I say does not agree with their preconceived ideas. So they do everything I say, except what I actually do say."

Holy Ceremony

A STUDENT who came to the lectures of a teacher, but had not become a disciple, was sometimes invited to stay on a little. On one occasion he asked about a Tantrik ceremony he had heard about. A pair, male and female, perform a rite on the night of the full moon, by which their sexual conjugation is sanctified and made uplifting. "I and my girlfriend have heard about this and we should like to try it. It seems a beautiful idea."

The teacher replied, "These things are not recognized in the classical tradition; they very rarely lead to any lessening of bondage to the world, with its consequent suffering."

But the student persisted that it was surely wrong to rule out any aspect of the divine current. He had been impressed with the phrase that in the ceremony, heaven and earth were made one.

Finally the teacher told him, "I have not practised these things, but I have read one of the principal texts. It is true that there are code-words in the texts: for instance, wine may be referred to by the word *tirtha*, literally meaning a holy place. But some participants have described them to me. In these rites, a principle of nature is solemnly worshipped with flowers and incense. A few sips of wine are permitted, but there must be no trace of vulgarity. The pair worship the divine principle in each other, and in the universe. They must fast the day before the ceremony, and must not touch each other during the twenty-eight days leading up to it."

The student was taken aback. "Wha-a-t? Oh, we couldn't do that. We thought this was just a special event once a month, a sort of extra. We can't let it interfere with our ordinary life."

The teacher gave a little smile. "Yes, some of the enthusiasts for these things somehow overlook plain statements of the text. They just pick out the things they think they will like. This Tantrik ceremony represents a restriction, not a license. Perhaps it was devised for people normally tending to be promiscuous. It requires tremendous strength of will; some of them call themselves heroes. They have to worship the divine principle with the same joy not only in some particular expression but when it strikes their body with accident or disease. These are no fair-weather worshippers, my friend. It is not impossible that there should be a spiritual benefit from such teaching, but there is a great risk of misunderstanding and abuse. That is one reason why it is not part of the classical tradition of the Upanishads and Gita, and it is best avoided."

Handshake

"I THINK it's wrong to avoid situations of temptation," declared a pupil somewhat positively. "If you do, it means you're afraid of them, and to fear them gives them power over you. It's neurotic. Of course one shouldn't seek them out, but if they come—well, let them come."

Others demurred. "We are told not to go voluntarily into places where we shall be tempted; in the Lord's Prayer too we pray not to be brought into temptation." There was no agreement, and they decided to put the point to a senior of long experience.

She said, "When one is still weak after an illness, it's a mistake to go out into a gale. It's not a question of being afraid; it's recognizing that one may not be able to keep one's footing in a sudden blast. Now we here are in the process of recovering from the illness of ignorance-of-the-Self. Most of us are convalescing; we are still weak. We recognize that we might not be able to keep our footing in a gale of old associations or new temptations. So we don't go out in them unnecessarily, until our legs are strong enough. Nothing wrong with that."

"But some of us are in circumstances where we can't avoid such things, however much we might like to," persisted the original objector, trying to save something of his point. "For instance, I'm occasionally in a position to swindle the firm out of money, which they couldn't trace."

"Our teacher said that it is best to arrange that someone is with you on those occasions; then there's no temptation. But that is not the final answer, it's true."

"What is the answer then?"

The senior stood up, and asked him to shake hands with her, and then hold on. They shook hands in the ordinary way. Then she said, "Now try to pull me across to you. And I'll try to stop you." She braced her feet, but the pupil was much stronger, and he easily pulled her to him. "Now try again," and she held out her hand. He took it as before and began to pull. But this time the hand was quite limp; it slipped from his grasp. He caught it again, and the same thing happened.

"You're not shaking hands properly," he said.

"No," she replied, "and so you had nothing firm to pull at. You can't get much purchase on something quite limp. It's difficult to carry away an unconscious man: Experts say it's easier if he's resisting a bit, because then his limbs are stiff. You can use them to lift him off his feet and then carry him.

"Well, when we meet temptations, we should try not to shake hands with them. To shake hands is to give them something firm to pull on. If we let ourselves get interested in them, or form pictures of them, then we are spiritually shaking hands. If we are alert, we can just drop the interest; it's not a question of effort, but dropping effort. If we have practised yoga, it's relatively easy to withdraw the vitality into the central line of the body. Then there's no clutching at the outer objects. They may momentarily take our hand, so to speak, but it will be quite slack, and they can't pull us to them.

"After a few experiences, we begin to feel the thrill of real independence."

Prescriptions

A TOUGH elderly pupil, once a well-known athlete in his youth, remarked on the calm rationality of the spiritual directions given by Vedanta, as against the fanatical emotionalism of some devotional sects.

"The instructions given us are like a doctor's prescriptions. I think Sankara says that somewhere. The suffering is analyzed, the cause is shown, and the patient is shown how to avoid it. Only if he fails to follow the preventive advice does treatment have to be applied.

"It's a very fine way to tackle spiritual illness to treat it on the same lines as physical illness. My own doctor, as a matter of fact, sometimes comes out with things which just fit both cases. Only the other day he said to me, 'Look, do you *want* to get ill? No? Then take my advice now. Don't wait till you get ill and then come and ask me to cure you.'"

"And what was he telling you to do?"

"Oh, that. Well, that was a bit ridiculous, as a matter of fact. He wanted me to begin wearing long thick underclothes. He said I mustn't get cold.

"But I told him straight out that I've never worn underclothes in my life and I'm not going to begin now. If it comes to that, I've never worn a top hat in my life either, but I don't have to start going round in one now, just because I'm a bit older. Why should I change my style of dress just because he says so? I don't criticize the way he dresses, though I could. I certainly could. But I don't. I leave his dressing style alone, and he can leave mine alone. That's all I ask. Still, he comes out with some good ones sometimes. He was saying that he's much worse off than a faith healer, because the faith healer's patients at least believe in him, whereas his own patients expect him to heal them though they don't believe a word he says. I wrote that one down, so I wouldn't forget it."

Excuses

"I CAN'T be expected to practise yoga much," complained a pupil, "because I am now so busy with the final structure of my business. If I don't do that, it might begin to decline, and if that set in, it might even collapse. This is an exceptional time for me. Once the business is completely, firmly established, I'll be able to concentrate on yoga."

"It will never be completely, firmly established," replied the teacher. "Nothing in the world can be. Your present time of life is not exceptional, it's typical.

"After all, when one is a child, one can't practise yoga because one has never heard of it. Then at school or as an apprentice, or learning from mother about running a home— those are full-time, aren't they? Because one's learning new things all the time. Then in the romantic tides of youth, there's hardly the inclination to practise yoga. Then one is building up a trade, or bringing up the children: no time there. After retirement, and when the children have left, one's somehow a bit tired. One thinks, 'Well, I couldn't succeed in yoga even in the full strength of youth and then maturity: what chance have I got now when my energies are waning?'

"It's a train of excuses, from beginning to end. It's based on the wrong idea that yoga is adding a few more obligations and concerns to the existing ones. It is not. It is learning to withdraw at fixed times, and later at will, from the whirl of compulsive reactions. It's learning to lay things down, not simply taking up more and more.

"Beginners at anything are usually tense all the time, because they cannot yet understand which things are important and which are not. The expert knows how to relax, and when he can relax. So even apart from technical skill, his actions are more efficient.

"All the stages of life have advantages and disadvantages. The small child asks the great questions, which the parents cannot answer: he usually gets discouraged and gives them up. The energy of youth is an advantage, but may dissipate itself in what are later found to have been trivialities. Middle age often gives some stability, but also some little authority, and it can become possessiveness and petty domination. The fourth quarter of life is said by Manu to be specially favorable for the attempt to be spiritually free; the responsibilities have been discharged, and apparently compelling ties have loosened. But all too often, older people have let themselves turn into mere bundles of habits.

"We should look at the advantages of the stage of life we are in, and avoid making excuses. However much we pile up excuses, we shall find ourselves at the end without the great excuse."

"Why, what is that great excuse?"

"We shall find we have no excuse for having been born."

Test Not

IN A country where several religions were practised, including Christianity and Buddhism, a spiritual group existed which taught methods of mind-control and meditation without restrictions of belief. Believers found their own faith intensified by the practices, and were not asked to convert to a new faith.

They began to prosper, and undertook small charitable works where they saw a need. But these were to be occasions for practise of universality and serenity, not ends in themselves.

They were near a small school. Some of the children came from a distance on bicycles, which they had nowhere to put against the rain. It was proposed that the group offer to provide a little shed for them. The school, short of funds, gladly accepted. Two of the Outer Activities Committee, one a Buddhist and one a Christian, were appointed to see it done.

There was an elderly professional carpenter in the group, but he was not much liked by some because of his directness. Moreover, as he usually spoke only what he knew, he was often annoyingly right. So the Committee members asked two absolutely inexperienced members to do the job. This caused some surprise, and to justify their decision they said to a senior, "It is essential, don't you think?, that younger members get experience in this sort of do-it-yourself job. Of course we do have a carpenter, but that's no reason why he should automatically be called in. If he thought he was indispensable, it might lead to egoism. To have to stand down sometimes is a good test for him."

"This is going to affect others," replied the senior, "namely the children of the school. Our young people can get experience on things that don't affect the world outside."

"Ah, but then they would not feel responsible. They'd know it didn't really matter, and might be tempted to do it carelessly. It wouldn't be real experience."

"We are supposed to be training here to do things properly, once we have taken them on. Well, think it over. Because the same divine nature is in all of us, it doesn't follow that all of us express it equally well through shed-building. Still, you've been appointed, and you must make the decision."

The Committee members discussed it, but did not change their mind, and the two young ones began to build the shed. They had been told not to consult anyone, but simply to do their best. This they did, but soon the little shed began to leak, and then to tilt dangerously. The children stopped using it. The carpenter went to the school and offered to build a new one, free of charge. He made it firm and beautiful, which was criticized by some as egoistic self-display, though others thought it was just professional skill. The children used it from then on.

Soon afterwards, the original shed collapsed. That day there was a tacit agreement not to mention the embarrassing fact. Very early next morning the two Committee members got a cart and went quietly to take away the ruins, hoping to escape notice. On the way back, however, they encountered the senior sweeping the steps of their own centre.

The Buddhist said, with elaborate calm, "Everything changes. The Buddha-nature is change, and change should be welcome."

The senior straightened up and looked across toward the new shed, bright in the early sun: "Welcome indeed."

The Buddhist reddened, and looked away.

"All that happens is the will of God," added the Christian defiantly. "It must be the will of God, or it couldn't happen. Let

His will be done—it's all in the Bible."

"Yes, the Bible covers everything, doesn't it. Or nearly everything."

They could not be sure, but as they moved off they thought they heard a muttered, "Test not, lest ye be tested."

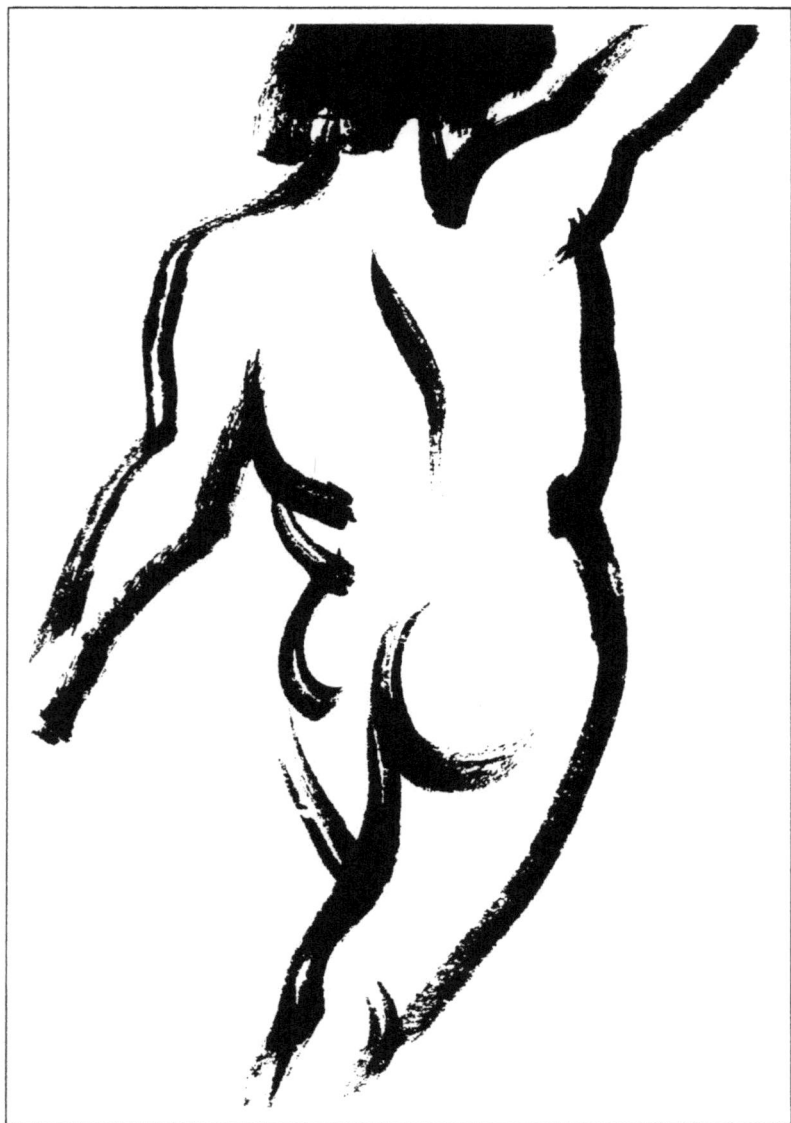

Giving Up Illusion

A YOUNG student was considering becoming a brahmacharin celibate for three years. The teacher told him that when combined with the yoga practices, it would give increased intelligence, energy, happiness, and inner serenity.

"You cannot just say no: it must be part of the system of disciplined practice."

It happened that the class was reading the Yoga Sutras of Patanjali, and they came to a passage picturing temptations that the brahmacharin has to be able to face. "Here is a girl so beautiful that she seems to have been carved out of the moon, whose glances light up the world wherever she looks, whose lips are honey," and so on. Afterwards he sought the teacher. "I doubt if I could give up a girl like that," he confessed.

"You are not asked to," replied the teacher. "This is a fantasy. Girls do not seem carved out of the moon; their lips are not honey. You are asked only to give up the fantasy."

"But there are girls—well, not perhaps exactly like that, but just as attractive. And I am being asked to give them up."

"You are not giving them up at all," rejoined the teacher, "assuming what you say, and that you might meet such a girl. You are asked to give up not her but the illusion that someone like you or I could hold the attention of a beauty like that even for a minute."

Fire Stages

AN INDIAN tradition says that training is usually like setting fire to wood that is a bit damp in places. It is difficult to get a flame at all, and it keeps going out. When it does catch hold a bit, great clouds of dense smoke arise, nearly choking the fire-raisers.

Then it begins to burn briskly, and people can benefit from the light and heat. Then it roars in triumph as the whole pile blazes.

Finally it dies down into the peace of the ashes.

In the Courtyard

THE CARPENTER was poor, and one day asked his spiritual teacher whether it was right to pray for a better living.

"I too am poor," said the teacher, "but after all I have a place to sleep and some food to eat, which some people have not. I am ashamed to ask the Lord for more when there are so many worse off than I am."

The carpenter thought resentfully, "But you have some rich disciples; why shouldn't they be asked to do something for me?" But he managed to remain silent. As the years went by, his reputation as a conscientious workman grew, and things improved, though only a little. He began to feel, however, a sort of peace in his heart, and no longer resented the better circumstances of others.

A new king came to the throne, energetic and efficient, and interested in spiritual things. Conditions generally improved. It was announced that the king was inaugurating a new scheme: one person out of each street would be chosen by lot, and invited to attend the palace to come before the king. Soon afterwards, a royal messenger told the carpenter that he was one of the lucky ones. The date and time were given to him.

He was passed through the great outer gate of the palace into a wide courtyard. On the other side was the inner door, guarded by a huge, magnificently attired guard with an impressive mustache. His right hand at the waist held upright a bare sword. Timidly the carpenter approached him and gave his name. The guard gestured toward a large tray on a stand,

"Put your presents there."

"'Presents'? I wasn't told about presents. How would someone like me have anything?"

The guard frowned. "No one goes in without making presents. Ministers, ambassadors, whoever they are, they all make presents. Put yours there. Put whatever you've got." He looked away.

The carpenter felt in his pocket, and found only three copper coins. They were hardly visible on the expanse of the tray. As he stood bewildered, his teacher came out of the door. Over his plain coat someone had hung strings of pearls; on his fingers were jeweled rings. He walked across and said, "I will arrange them for you."

As he bent to move the little coins about, the rings slipped off his fingers. The strings of the pearls broke, and they rained onto the tray in a cascade of light. The guard's eyes opened wide as the teacher carried the heaped-up tray past him into the palace.

Now, the carpenter's name was called from within, but he was too confused and ashamed to move; he stood looking down, twisting his toes in the dust. The guard crashed the sword into its scabbard, and strode across. Gently he slid his great hands under the little carpenter's armpits, and carried him bodily through the door.

"This is the last present," he said, "and the best."

Dream-Fair

IN THE dream I was in an old-style fair, like the fairs of my childhood: dazzling lights, blaring music, obscure comings and goings in the dark alleys between the stalls. The booths were selling Unhappiness, Failure, Disease, Disaster, Despair—all at high prices. I wandered around, and noticed a stall a little apart, with its shutters up. An inconspicuous notice read: "The Kingdom of the Universe: First Customer Only." I smiled and went on.

I lost my way, and later found myself before the little stall again. The front shutter was being taken down from inside, revealing a counter and dimly behind it a stalwart, fierce-looking old man in a patched cloak. He looked at me, and on impulse I put my little handful of money on the counter, but keeping back three coins which I knew I would need to get back home.

"You are the first customer!" cried the old man in an arresting voice which made some of the passing crowd stop and look. "But the bid is not enough. Are there any supporters?"

As if pulled by strings, some of the crowd came forward. A soldier put his bedizened sword on the counter beside my coins: "Remember me when you come to your greatness," he muttered. An old lady laid down a few trinkets. "These are my treasures, mementos of my dear husband. Remember me." A merchant put a bar of gold, and others brought jewels.

"Still not enough, not quite enough," shouted the stall-holder. "It wants three copper coins more to make up the price."

The others looked helplessly at each other. "We have given everything, we have no more," they whispered.

My hand felt the three little coins in my pocket, but I knew I needed them. I could not give these too.

"The price has not been met: I am going to close the shop!" The voice was like thunder. My hand still closed on the three coins. Patched-cloak raised his hand. There was dead silence. Time stopped. Nothing moved.

Was it only this once, or has it been many times, dream after dream, incarnation after incarnation, that I have stood there, clutching the last coins that I will not give up?

Fireworks

A YOGA pupil in Calcutta knew the manager of a theatre, and was sometimes presented with a free seat. On one such occasion he saw a demonstration of thought-reading; the manager said as he handed over the ticket, "This is in your line." The central part of the show was that the performer came to the front of the stage, opened his arms wide, and asked the audience each to think some question strongly. After a short time, he announced, "There is a lady in the fifth row, worrying about her mother, who has had a road accident. Her leg is broken. If this is correct, will the lady please stand up and acknowledge it? I can tell her that her mother will recover well."

A middle-aged woman stood up and said, "That is right. Thank you." The pupil assumed that she was a confederate of the thought-reader.

However, he decided on a little experiment of his own. His father was an import-export merchant dealing in commodities. So he concentrated on the jute market, in which he knew his father was interested. Will the price go up or down? To his surprise, the thought-reader said, a little later, "There is a young man inquiring about a particular commodity market. I can tell him the price will go up."

The pupil told his father. The next day, the jute market price did go up. The father insisted on going to the theatre the next evening, and got the manager to take him to the performer's dressing room. He asked him how much he earned with his thought-reading, and offered him five times that fee to advise him on the markets.

The man laughed, "My dear sir, if I could tell the future, do you think I would be here on the stage for these little fees? When I open my arms and stand there, I do pick up some thoughts, usually an anxiety. But as to answers—I have to make that up. That is one reason why I have to keep moving round the country—some of my guesses turn out rather badly."

The pupil told this to his spiritual teacher, who remarked, "Such things are like fireworks. They seem brilliant and impressive, but they are useless for life. You cannot read by the light of fireworks, you cannot cook or warm yourself by their fire, and they disappear almost at once. Those who try to develop them become inwardly restless, and very often take to alcohol to relieve the inner sense of strain. Sometimes a trace of such things comes unsought to a yogin, but to play with them means loss of independence, and can set back spiritual progress for incarnations. You can't get anything out of them at all.

"Tell your friend the theatre manager that such performances have nothing to do with spiritual training: in fact they impede it."

The pupil told the story to a British friend, who later encountered another case; the parallels are striking.

The head of a famous Japanese hospital was visiting Britain as delegate to a medical congress. He had been an expert in Judo, and found friends at the main London Judo club. As a side interest, he had done some investigation of the so-called psychic phenomena among Japanese *miko* (a sort of priest, often a woman); he said that he had on several occasions seen something like a star traveling across the shrine. "But (as he remarked) these are not controlled conditions. And it may be that controlled conditions upset the delicate balance of trance concentration. In which case such phenomena might never be fully established." Among the club members was a prominent British spiritualist, and at the doctor's request he arranged a séance with a reputed medium. Afterwards the doctor was rather thoughtful for a few days.

Then he was his usual cheerful self, and he said to the British captain of the Judo club, "You are a high-grade Judo man, and I pass this on to you privately. That medium told me a few generalities which might be true of many people. But she also told me correctly that I have four children, and she got their ages right. At the end of the sitting, she added, 'Oh yes, and your wife has cancer of the throat.'

"As a matter of fact, just when I was leaving, my wife did mention casually to me that she had a sore throat. I said I would look at it when I got back. But after hearing that medium, I sent a cable to my deputy to get my wife in immediately for an exploratory operation on the throat. I was uneasy for a couple of days—perhaps you noticed—and then I got the cable in reply: 'Your wife has a slight soreness of the throat.'

"I realized that the medium must have picked up that slight worry from my mind—I am a doctor, and my wife's remark must have registered as a remote anxiety. She picked that up, and then something decided to have a bit of fun with me, it seems. After establishing her credit with the children and their ages, it certainly worked."

The British captain thought, "Just like the witches in *Macbeth*." And he remembered what the Calcutta pupil had told him about the teacher's comment, "You can't get anything out of them at all."

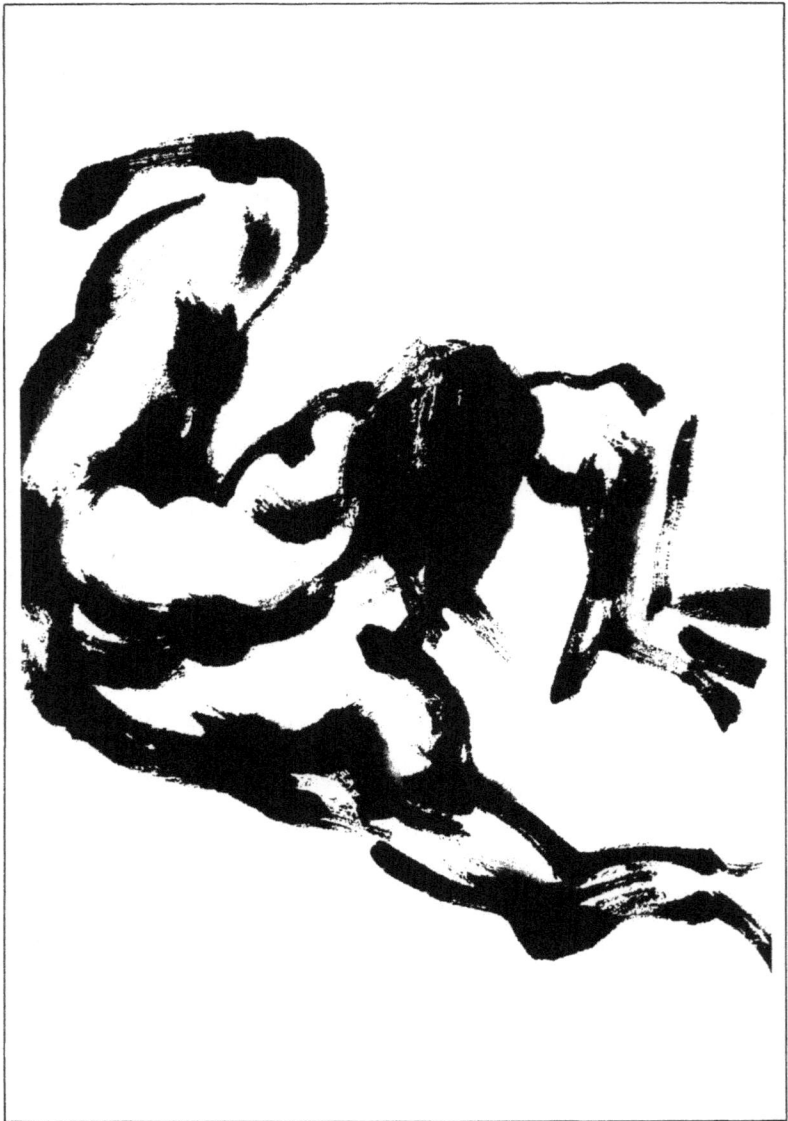

The Swimmer

AN ANXIOUS man, always trying to foresee every possible eventuality so that he could prepare countermeasures, came to a yoga group. There he took to reading up historical and legendary incidents in the scriptures, so that he would get to know how spiritual people behave.

"You've no need to do that," an experienced disciple told him. "Our teacher tells us to try to become enlightened ourselves, rather than just reading about the enlightenment and enlightened actions of others."

"But then how is one to know what to do?" replied the new disciple, and he went on as before.

He happened to be an expert swimmer, and the senior one day asked him whether he could demonstrate the racing dive he had heard about. The swimmer readily agreed, pleased to be able to show his skill, and they went together to the swimming baths. The expert changed into swimming trunks, and they walked together along the side of the baths toward the diving boards. The swimmer was on the side next to the water. Suddenly the other gave him a violent push, and he fell into the bath and went under. He came to the surface quickly, climbed out, and looked inquiringly at the senior, who said, "You went into the water sideways, in quite a tangle trying to recover your balance, didn't you? Have you ever gone into the water like that before?"

"Why no. Who would ever go in like that? Unless he was pushed, of course."

"Then how did you know what to do? You say you've never practised it. How is it that you could come up so quickly? I was ready to help in case you got into trouble, but you had no difficulty at all. What exactly did you do?"

The swimmer laughed. "I don't know exactly what I did. I just made the proper movements to come up—I don't know what they were. But of course I came up at once because I'm a swimmer. A swimmer would always come up quite easily; he doesn't have to practise that sort of thing, because he's a swimmer, he's a swimmer."

"In the same way you've no need to rehearse or practise for life's unexpected turns, if you're a yogi. You'll meet them in some proper way, because you're a yogi, you're a yogi."

Mistakes

A PUPIL who lived rather carelessly remarked, "Mistakes are a necessary part of the path of training. If you read the biographies of even the greatest, they all say that they made many mistakes. Some of them say that mistakes are a necessary part of the training—one learns from them. So I don't worry about my own conduct: Let the mistakes come, I think, let 'em all come. I'll go through them and come out the other side. It is all part of the path."

This was put to a senior pupil, a businesswoman, for her opinion. She remarked, "You need not tell him I said this, but I don't think our teacher would rate the idea very high in terms of clear thinking. It's easy to get woolly about spiritual things. I remember when I learned to type. It was in a class. Of course we made mistakes, but the teacher always stressed the importance of getting the habit of absolutely accurate typing. He never said that as mistakes are inevitable in learning to type, let 'em all come. He told us we should type very slowly, if necessary, to reduce the mistakes to almost nil. Those of us who followed his advice finally learned to type with perfect accuracy without thinking about it. The others, though at first they typed a bit quicker, were always subject to occasional lapses and never became good typists. Mistakes are like the falls when one is taking up skating. Some are inevitable, but we should make them as few as possible. They are part of the path, it is true, but they are stumbles, not forward steps."

Too Good

IN A thick grove some way outside the town was a small temple, looked after by a widowed retired businessman, who was a devotee of the divinity of the shrine. It was traditionally said, and widely believed, that anyone who came on foot to worship there, with a pure heart, every day for forty days, would receive blessings. Few undertook the forty days, but many people made occasional visits, and some of them experienced great relief from anxieties after the visit. They used to make a small donation according to their means to the temple each time they visited.

The temple keeper spent a good deal of his time washing it spotlessly clean, and polishing the surfaces to get them to shine. This was no easy matter, owing to the nature of the stone. He felt that the work he did was not appreciated by the worshippers who came and went; they saw him working, of course, but none of them realized how much he did.

He happened to notice that some birds had nested in a tree near the entrance to the path through the grove; when a visitor approached, these birds would call out to each other. One day when the birds suddenly became particularly noisy, he guessed that a group was coming, and immediately set to work energetically. As they came up they saw him furiously scouring the stone at the side of the temple (not near the door—he thought that would be too obvious). The little group of six performed their worship and left. It was part of the ritual to keep silent till they had got out of the grove, but he knew that then they would probably burst out into conversation. He ran along a little side-path and hid, so that he could overhear what was said.

Sure enough, one remarked, "Did you see that fellow working at the side wall? Terrific, wasn't it! He couldn't have known we were coming, either."

"He must have," retorted another contemptuously, "and it was all an act. He must have known we were coming somehow. How could he possibly keep that pace up? He was doing it too hard to be genuine, I'm afraid. Ham acting, not working, that was."

The devotee heard all his hopes punctured: he knew the story would go round. He felt a sense of futility, and began to do less work on the temple. But the inner bitterness did not lessen. Ham acting, ham acting, ham acting. Lazy swine, he thought, what do any of them do? Sometimes he would see the pointlessness of his circling thoughts, and almost overcome them, but then the suppressed fury would blaze up again.

In desperation he spent a whole night in self-examination, praying for light. Enlightenment comes with the dawn, he had heard somewhere. As dawn came, he realized, not merely intellectually but in his heart, that he had been cleaning the temple not as a service for the god, but for the good opinion of worshippers. He was able to work again, but quietly now, with his mind centred on service to heaven, without thought of men. After forty days he noticed a calm spreading outward from his heart throughout his body and movements. As he grew older, his body worked more slowly, but the peace grew deeper and deeper.

One day as he was polishing in the sunlight, a voice behind him said, "Sir." He turned and saw a group of young people looking at him with interest and respect. The man who had spoken, whom he had seen a few times at the temple, continued, "My cousin from a long way off came on a visit, and I brought him here. He is master of a stonemason's business, and told me that this stone is very difficult to polish. When he heard that it is only a single man who looks after the whole temple, he told us that it is a great work of service that has been done here. We had not realized it; we thought the stone shone naturally. With your permission, I and my friends would like to help you, under your direction."

A couple of helpers dropped away in time, but the others remained, and new ones joined. After a year, one of them said to the old man, "Sir, I have noticed that your movements are smooth, and you do not seem to get tired. Would you tell me something about this? We get tired, though we are young."

"Why," he said, "I have been doing this for a long time. No doubt I am used to it."

"Surely that is not all, is it, sir?"

The old man looked into the sincere face in front of him, and said slowly, "My work has changed. At first I used to think of the Maurya stone near where I once lived. It is beautifully polished, and has kept its sheen for over two thousand years. I thought I would polish the temple like that; it would be a wonderful achievement and everyone would admire it. I was worshipping myself as I worked. Then I began to hanker after some appreciation."

He told him the story of the visiting group, and the sarcastic remark about ham acting. "I had been worshipping the opinions of others. But then I began to be able to work simply to serve the Lord who is enshrined here."

"How do you see our work, sir?"

"What are you thinking of as you work?"

The man pondered. "Well, when I am polishing one bit, I suppose I am thinking that I should get this really shining, and then move on to the next bit, and I have a vague idea of how many days it will take to finish the whole wall. And that will be my offering to the Lord."

"While you think like that you will get tired. I do not say it is bad, but you will get tired."

"Then how do you do it, sir?"

"I polish the bit that is in front of me, without thinking of anything else. As I polish it, I am polishing my heart. And then ... I realize that the Lord is polishing my heart. And then ... I realize that the Lord is polishing the wall."

He stopped. There was a silence. "And is there anything else, sir?"

In a very low voice, the old man whispered, "Sometimes I think I see the Lord reflected dimly in the polished wall."

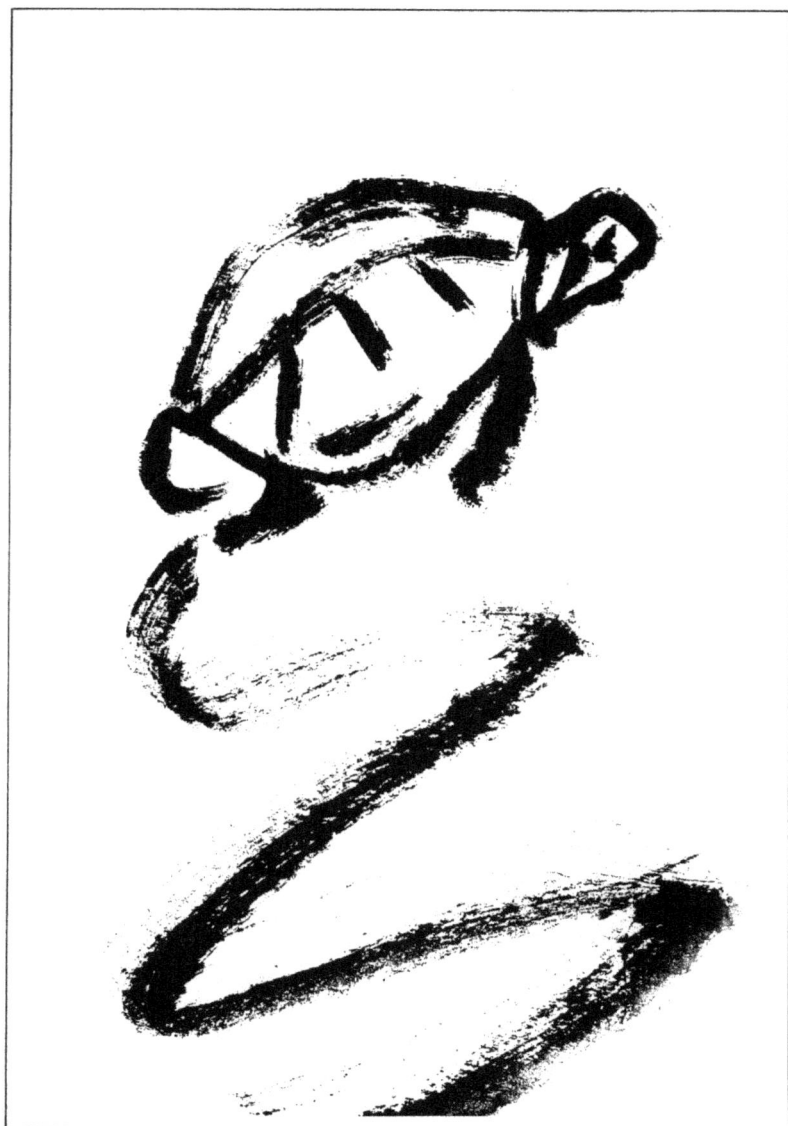

Turtle

DISCIPLES nearly always pass through a phase when they feel that it is no use doing any service to the spiritual group or to fellow men, no use in fact doing anything with a purpose, because all these things will reinforce egoity, the feeling "I am doing it."

They may drop for quite a long time into a sort of inertia, thinking, "Well now, at any rate I am not being *egoistic.*"

To a pupil in this state a teacher told a parable:

"It is a tradition in ancient China that the turtle smoothes out its footsteps in the mud by wiping them out with its tail as it goes along. It leaves no footmarks, and therefore its enemies cannot follow its footsteps.

"But the enemies follow the marks left by the tail."

"Then what is one to do?" wondered the pupil.

"You cannot stamp out your egoity, but you can forget it. Forget yourself in the action; perform your actions without hoping for a result or fearing the results of failure. Perform the actions for the joy of the movement itself; feel the natural impulse to beauty and order flowing through your movements and actions. Do not think of what went before or what may come after, but lose yourself in this which has come before you. You will feel as if you had been relieved of an awkward and hampering burden, and your actions will become light."

One Step, Twenty Steps

"WHEN SOMEONE takes one step toward the Lord, the Lord takes twenty steps toward him." It is a striking phrase which has vivified and energized the devotion of many yogis. Nevertheless, it can be interpreted, disregarding the plain meaning of the words, into something quite different. In a lazy period, one who believes himself a devotee can reason something like this:

> What this says is that when I take a step toward him, the Lord takes twenty steps toward me. In fact he is doing the same as I do, namely taking one step, and then he adds nineteen more of his own. So if I take no step at all, then admittedly the Lord will not take that step either; but then he will add nineteen steps of his own to it. Adding nineteen to nothing gives nineteen, so he will still move nineteen steps toward me. He won't arrive quite so quickly, perhaps, but the difference will soon be made up.

Someone who heard of this remarked, "That idea is based on addition, and it is against the clear meaning. What the text says is that when one step is taken toward the Lord, the Lord multiplies it by twenty. Even if it is only a single step, that step of the devotee becomes twenty steps by the Lord. But if the devotee cannot be bothered to take even one step ... well, twenty times nothing is nothing. It is true that the Lord could appear immediately, but he leaves it to a devotee to have the joy of himself coming, even a little, toward the Lord."

Warning

THERE WAS a discussion about whether it is necessary, or even right, to give a warning on a spiritual matter when it is clear that it will not be heeded at all. One view was that in such cases it is meaningless, and the instance was given of a saintly man who had given a warning about the sin of using violence to a crowd of self-styled patriots. Their response was to beat him, and then go on with their program, which in the event led to the calamities for others and themselves which he had predicted.

A member of the sangha asked for an explanation. "Did that saintly man know they wouldn't listen? Or did he simply miscalculate?"

"Nothing is absolutely impossible, and he would have been following a spiritual impulse to speak out," said a senior, "but, yes, he would have known that in the ordinary course they would never listen to him."

"Then why do it?" persisted the other. "The Gita says yoga is skill in action. Surely it isn't skillful action to waste the breath like that, and provoke them as well."

"I used to think so too, but then I had an experience of it from the other side. And that made me change my mind. I was very ambitious when I was young, and I suddenly got a good chance to make a jump in my career. I knew that one of the other sangha members had had something similar a little time before. To my amazement, however, an old and rather tottery sangha member approached me, and timidly hinted that I should be careful about taking up anything that would excite ambition. I guessed that this came indirectly from the teacher, but I brushed it aside with one sharp comment about interference. I assumed this was some sort of routine warning given mechanically to pupils. But my opinion of the teacher's insight went down a bit; there was not the faintest possibility of my listening to that sort of thing, particularly through that sort of intermediary. (At that time I couldn't distinguish between a letter and the postman.)

"As things turned out, my project was successful. But it did cause me a good deal of anxiety. I found I couldn't stop thinking about it; it invaded my thoughts and hindered my yoga practice. It was a long time before I could get free.

"When I look back on the beginning and end of that time of self-created difficulty, one thing stood out clearly: I had been warned. There had been no possibility of my listening, but ... I had been warned. And that gave me confidence in the teacher. From then on, I paid great respect to what he said. If he had not given that warning, futile though it seemed to be at the time, it might have taken much longer to get on a firm basis.

"It may well be that some of those terrorists too will look back and realize: We were warned."

Hypnosis

Question: Is there any benefit to be gained from using methods like self-hypnosis as an aid to meditation?

Answer: None at all. In self-hypnosis some elements of the personality are put to sleep, so to say. But they are not changed. Suppose there is a family whose house needs painting but we cannot agree on what colour it should be painted. We all feel strongly about it, so it does not get painted at all. Now I think, "I should like the house painted green, but they will not agree." I give my relatives a drug which sends them to sleep, and while they are snoring I paint the house green. I have, in a sense, hypnotized them, and got my idea through.

But when they wake up ... !

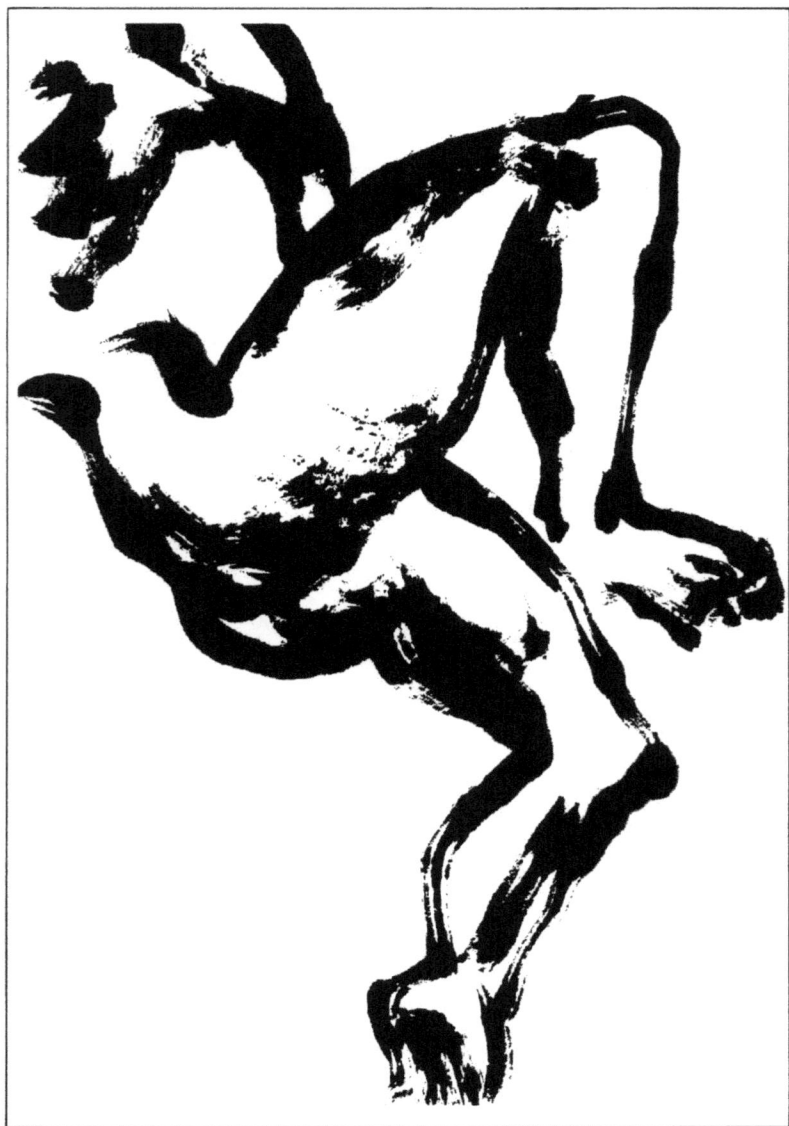

The Procession

A GREAT mahatma (Rama Tirtha) after his realization found he could no longer continue a home life in society, as professor of mathematics (at Lahore University). He went to live at great heights in the Himalayas, occasionally coming down to give talks and publish articles. On one such occasion his former teacher sent a young disciple to look after him.

One day the mahatma gave a four-hour-long discourse to an audience of thousands; he danced on the sands of the Ganges, and many of the audience saw a god there dancing.

Afterwards he went back with the young brahmachari to the small room where he was staying. The mahatma's lack of interest in food, and his solitary life in the mountains, had upset his digestive system, and he sometimes suffered from attacks of colic. When the spasms came on, his body twisted and turned. The disciple watched this with horror, and when he found there was nothing he could do to help, he burst into tears.

The mahatma patted him on the head and said to him, "My son, Rama is above all this."

"But when you danced, we saw a god dancing there," sobbed the brahmachari, "and now this. How can this happen to you?"

The mahatma replied, "You know the procession of Rama when it goes through the village, don't you? What a joyous occasion it is! The image of the god passes, so majestic, so exalting; then the band and its music, and some of the devotees singing the songs of divine love. Then there are the acrobats, who follow the palanquin of the god, displaying their skill to take part in this great occasion. And finally there are the clowns, aren't there? They turn somersaults to amuse the children and to add to the general happiness. You know all this, and you appreciate it all.

"The same thing is happening here—it is a divine procession through the body of Rama. The dance on the sands—that was the passing of the god before your eyes. And now, following the procession, here are the acrobats and the clowns, making their bodies twist and turn. It is all the divine procession—and Rama is an onlooker, appreciating it."

The Well

SOME STUDENTS discourage themselves by looking at themselves each day. After trying hard for a session, they feel that as there has been no result they have failed.

Next day they try again, and again they fail. Gradually this builds up into a conviction of continuous failure, and they begin to think, "Oh, what's the use of trying?"

For such occasions there is an ancient Indian example, that of the well-digger.

The Indian tradition was that beneath the desert there is water, however deeply hidden. This has recently been confirmed in the case of the vast Rajasthan desert in northwest India, beneath which a legendary river was supposed to flow. It has been established that the river is actually there though deep underground.

The maxim of the well-digger is this: Each day when he digs but finds no water, he does not think, "I have failed." Next day he digs again, deeper, and so on day after day. Every evening, though he has found no water yet, he thinks not, "I have failed," but "Nearer, nearer, nearer!"

Dragon Pool

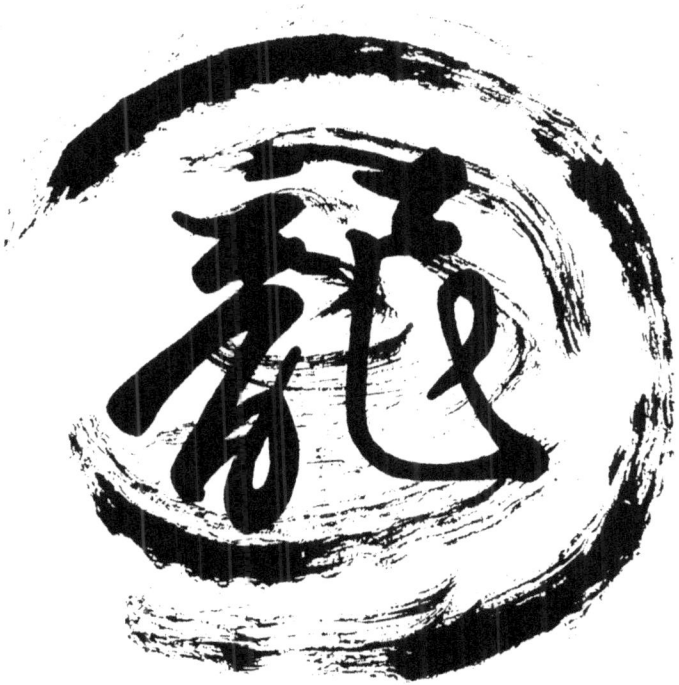

Remembering

A WOMAN disciple had been told—as all the disciples were told—to choose one verse from a holy text each week, and learn it by heart. She protested to a senior, for whom she had a great respect, "That would be quite impossible for me. Even as a child I have never been able to memorize things."

"How do you know?" asked the senior.

"Why, at one of my first classes in infant school, we were set to learn a little list by heart: it was six dates, and the others learned them quite quickly. But I just couldn't. I couldn't. And at the end of the lesson, the school mistress (I can see her now, in her black bombazine and jet bracelets, all sweetness on the surface but hard as nails underneath) said that the others could go home but I was to sit there till I had learned it. Well, I couldn't learn it. We just sat there: me, and her looking at me, with her lips in a straight line. After an hour, my mother came to find where I was, and when she learned what had happened she took me away. That's how I know I can't remember things."

"You seem to remember that pretty well," remarked the senior, and she suddenly blazed up with some wounding remarks about deliberate idiocy angling for special treatment, not stopping at offensive personal remarks.

The junior went out almost in tears. She stayed away for several days, and then came back obviously uncertain of her reception.

The senior greeted her most kindly, and after a little conversation said, "You seem a bit pensive—is anything the matter?"

"Oh, no, nothing," replied the disciple reproachfully. "Only what you said to me the other day."

"Why, what did I say?"

"You said that, and then you said that, and then ..." and the disciple recounted the cutting slights point by point.

"So you can remember, then? How is it that you can remember all that, and yet you can't remember one little verse from the holy texts?"

"Because that applied to me. The texts don't apply to me personally; they're declarations of the holy truth, I suppose, but they don't apply to me personally."

"Ah," said the senior. "That's where you might be wrong, you know. All that nonsense I was talking doesn't apply to you at all—it just applied maybe to some clown whom you let into your role for a moment. But the holy texts apply to you, to the real you.

"Apply them to yourself, to yourself personally, as clearly and sharply as you applied those silly remarks of mine, then you'll find you can remember the verses easily."

Reverence

A DEVOUT pupil attended a spiritual meeting in another part of the country, at which holy texts were intoned by individual men and women.

On his return he told his teacher that he had been shocked by the lack of reverence shown by those reciting the texts. "I had heard that they were a very good group, but they did not seem to show respect for what they were reading. You have told us that we should always read holy texts with great reverence."

The teacher, who was well known for deep insight, asked, "And did you feel the truth of the texts when they were being recited as you say?"

"Why, yes. It was very clear and firm. But no reverence—that put me off."

The teacher said, "When we recite the holy texts, we must always do it with great reverence. But if it should come to pass that there is no more 'I' or 'we,' then there is no reverence either. The holy texts speak out the truth as it is: they have nothing to do with reverence or no reverence. That's for human beings who still feel themselves separate individuals."

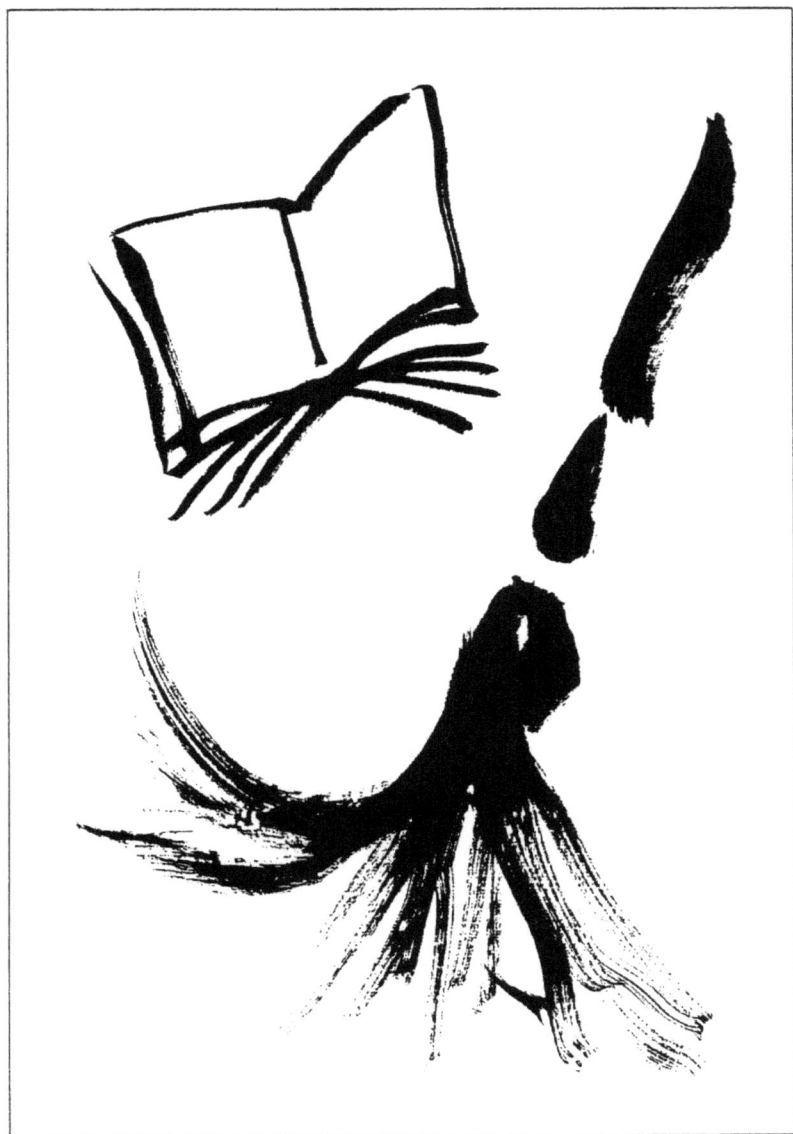

Humble

THE TEMPLE had a good number of rare manuscripts, and the librarian, an excellent scholar, catalogued them efficiently and arranged for their publication. Scholars came to consult him from distant centres of learning, and the temple and its librarian became famous.

One day a visitor was congratulating him on his great contributions to learning, and the priest looked out of the window and pointed to an old man sweeping up the leaves in the garden.

"That is a humble task," he said with a very kindly smile. "And people sometimes forget that the library, and the whole temple in fact, is supported on humble work like that, humble work like that. In their own way, he and others like him make a great contribution."

The visitor was impressed, and when he said farewell to the abbot he mentioned the incident. "When I saw that humble man sweeping up the leaves," he said, "and listened to such kind words about him by that wonderful scholar the librarian, I realized the unity of the temple for the first time."

"Oh, he's not exactly humble," answered the abbot. "He's thinking that although the librarian is so famous and he himself is unknown outside this temple, still when the spiritual truth comes out (and if he has anything to do with it, it soon will), it will be the simple gardener who is acclaimed, and the arrogant librarian who is humiliated. And in the meantime, he gives the assistant gardener hell.

"Both those two have some way to go before they realize that becoming famous as a librarian and sweeping the leaves in the garden are spiritually the same thing. They are occasions for practise and ultimately illumination and inspiration; the outward form of the occasion has no importance at all.

"The Buddha-wind is turning the leaves in the library through the fingers of the librarian, and turning the leaves in the garden through the broom of the gardener, but it is not the same Buddha-wind."

Racing Dive

A WELL-KNOWN modern Zen master, on tour with his attendant, visited a Zen centre for lay folk founded by a pupil of his. In addition to their sitting practice, they were encouraged to undertake joint social work to help the local school and so on, but not so much that it became an overriding concern.

When he was introduced to the members, the master seemed to have an immediate understanding with one of the women, a longtime member of the group. She was known as a good quiet worker, but not otherwise remarkable. He did not give her special attention, though he asked her opinion on several points. When the time came for the individual farewells, the two of them stood for a few seconds looking into each other's eyes. The head of the group took the opportunity to thank the master for his "kindness, to each one of our humble lay group. It is an example of the Buddhist principle of No Distinctions," he concluded. "No distinctions indeed," agreed the master, and she repeated, "No distinctions." They burst out laughing, bowed to each other, and then both bowed to the slightly confused group leader. The little occasion was over.

On the way home, the attendant found himself wondering about what he had seen. On return, he was asked by a senior how it had gone, and related the incident. He then asked whether the master had seen something special in that lay follower, and if so, by what indications. "A trained eye can see much more than an untrained one," replied the senior, "but usually such indications can't be explained." The attendant persisted, and finally the other said, "Well, I'll tell you a case from another field."

"When I was young I was interested in sport, and a student friend, a first-rate swimmer, offered to give me advanced lessons. When I was tired, I sat for a rest on the side of the bath while my friend swam up and down. I saw a very athletic-looking man come out of the changing rooms and stand on the edge of the bath, obviously waiting for a little clearing so that he could dive in. Looking at his trained physique, and posture straight as a spear, I thought, 'Now we'll see something.'

"My friend happened to swim up then, and beckoned me to come in. I told him, 'I just want to see this chap go in.' He just glanced across and said, 'He's no good. Come on in.' And so it proved: the athlete had clearly not trained at swimming.

"Afterwards when I asked how he had known, he said, 'Oh, he had his feet together. If you dive off from that position, the body will twist a bit, and the first stroke will be impaired. In a race that might be decisive. The racing dive is always made with the feet underneath the shoulders; then there's no twist.'

"I objected, 'But he wasn't in a race then ...'"

"No, but once you've learned the racing dive, you never again have the feet together. Even just standing around in the baths, you'd never want anything to do with that horrible twist. Under the shoulders—that's where your feet would be."

"I've given you that example: now as to our master, of course I can only guess. Both of them were then functioning in distinctions—place and time, Zen master and lay worker, man and woman, and all the rest. But perhaps when they met, they saw something in each other of an inner posture ready at any time for a racing dive into No-distinctions. The spiritual feet were under the spiritual shoulders. And no horrible twist."

Devil, Devil

THERE IS a method of reciting certain sutras, or parts of sutras, in which special attention is put on to the sound uttered. The would-be reciter sometimes practises for a time in the open, intoning the sonorous Chinese monosyllables into the wind on the edge of a cliff, or against the roar of a waterfall.

If all goes well, gradually he comes to feel that he is bringing out all his insides with the utterance, and that his voice is penetrating the whole scene before him. It is technically called "reciting the sutra with the whole body." When he can realize the feeling, he practises to retain it even when he repeats the sutra very softly. He still feels his body one with the sound, and syllables resonating with the universe.

It can take a long time to acquire skill in this practise, and some of those who do might certainly have reason to feel pleased with themselves.

One of the lesser-known sutras is thought to be particularly suited to this practice, and a city businessman, a practitioner of the method, having heard about it, asked his teacher to coach him in it.

He took as his exercise to do one long chapter every evening before retiring. He made this an invariable rule, and was determined never to break it, a vow which he had communicated to the teacher.

One day his company sent him to look at a stretch of remote coastline which they were considering developing as a part of a larger operation. The only human habitation was a village, and he had to stay overnight at the one small inn. He successfully made the inspection for the company, but when he unpacked his night things in the evening, he was horrified to find that by some mischance he had failed to bring his copy of the sutra. He did not know it by heart, and he asked the innkeeper whether he could borrow a copy. But it turned out that the innkeeper did not himself have anything but the usual Lotus Sutra, and the village temple was closed, the priest being away. In confusion, he resolved to telephone the teacher and ask him what to do. There was only one telephone in the little inn, and he had to make the call from the host's own room. As he sat in a corner, explaining the situation, he noticed that the host was talking to another guest, a handsome intelligent-looking man with an arrogant expression. They went on with their conversation, but obviously they were bound to hear everything he said, and he thought he saw a look of contempt on the face of the guest.

The teacher told him over the telephone, "You must accept this as it has happened; it must have a meaning for you. Now do not attempt your recitation, but instead recall as much as you can of the meaning of the sutra. Do not think of the sounds but of what the World-Honored One meant his listeners to understand."

"But I have always been reciting this for the sound; my practise will have lost its point. Of course I suppose the meaning is important, but this sutra is very fitted for the repetition by sound: you said so yourself. How could the Buddha want that I should not do it now?"

"Well, when the Buddha first gave this sutra, the listeners went by the meaning. He wasn't saying it in Chinese. And the Buddha is telling you now that tonight you too should go deeply into the meaning."

"'Deeply into the meaning'? I remember some of it, of course, but I don't know that I ..." and his voice trailed off.

Somewhat crushed, the reciter stammered out his thanks

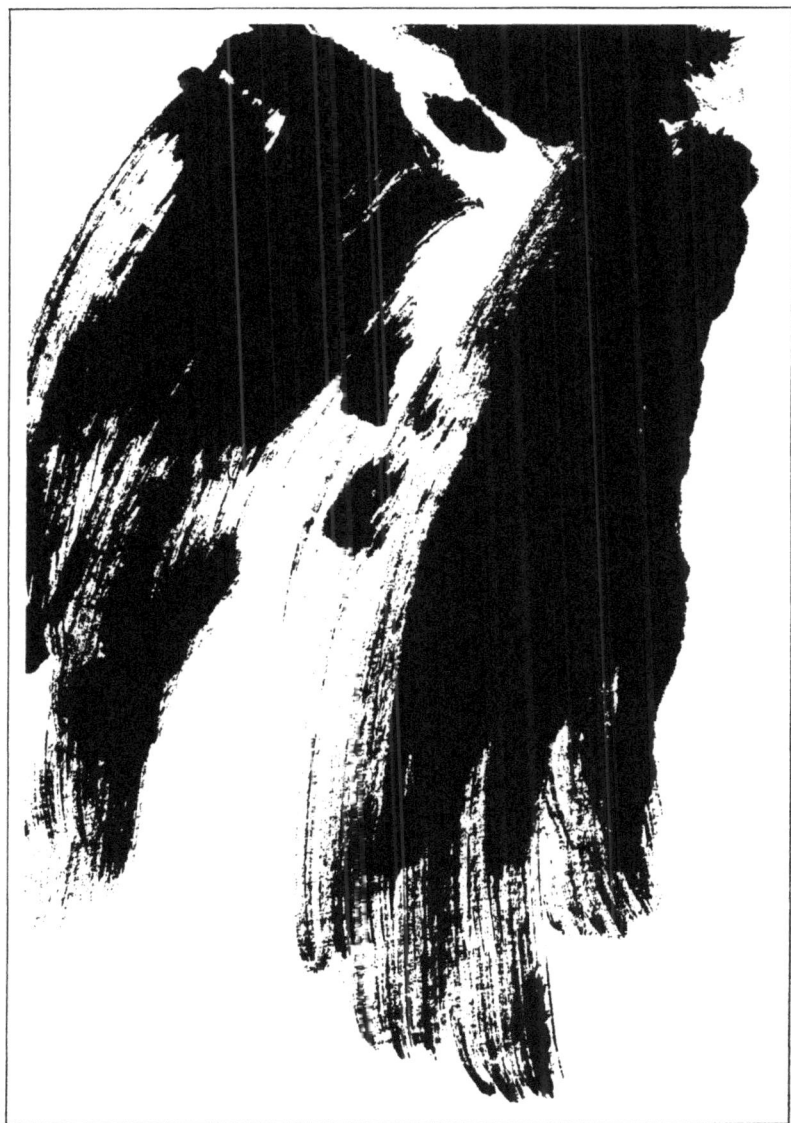

and put the phone down slowly. At the same time he noticed the other guest get up abruptly and go out.

He had his evening meal alone in his room, still trying to think of some way round the difficulty, as he hoped he would not have to follow the teacher's second-best method. When the maid was taking away the tray, a voice from outside said, "Excuse us—may we come in for a moment?" It was the host and the handsome man.

The latter approached him respectfully with a small book wrapped up in silk. He said, "I hope you will excuse my impertinence, but I could not help overhearing a bit of your conversation on the telephone a little time ago. It so happens that my wife's sister in the village is a devout reciter of sutras, and it occurred to me that very possibly she might have a copy of the one you want, though I understand from what you said that it is not very widely known. Well, I ventured to go round to ask her, and by great good fortune it turned out that she did have one. I think she may have been a little surprised to hear me asking about it, but I explained your position, and she was most sympathetic. She is very willing to lend it to you for the evening; please just leave it with my good friend the host when you depart early tomorrow, as I suppose you will have to do. She says you are not to feel any sense of obligation; as a fellow devotee, she is honored to have the opportunity of offering a little help."

The businessman was overwhelmed with gratitude, and thanked him profusely.

The kindly guest then took his leave. As he went out he turned and looked at the devotee with a curious expression, which the latter could not interpret.

The host stayed behind to make sure that the man from the city had everything he needed. After confirming that all was satisfactory, he remarked, "It was most unexpected that he should go to all that trouble to find and bring you that sutra. He always says that Buddhism tends to make people lazy. In fact he is a fanatical opponent of Buddhism; his nickname is Yasha (devil). And he lives up to it, as far as Buddhism is concerned. He's dead against sutra-reading or anything like that. At least, that's what everyone thought. But perhaps that was wrong, at any rate in this case."

"Yes, he's certainly been an angel to me," remarked the city man.

"Well, I'm very glad. As a fellow member of our village, I'm proud that he wanted to show our hospitality regardless of personal beliefs," smiled the host, as he said good night and went out.

The devotee carefully unwrapped the copy of the sutra and placed it before him. But he found that he could not get out of his head what the teacher had said about the Buddha wanting him to go deeply into the meaning of the sutra instead of reciting it, and mixed up with that came the vision of the strange look which the benefactor had given at the end. He found that he could interpret that look now. It had been a look of triumph. This had been no kindly impulse, but a devil looking with satisfaction on something accomplished.

"Why has the devil brought me this sutra? Why is the yasha so pleased with what he has done?" Slowly he realized it all. That restless, intelligent mind had seen through his own self-satisfaction at his ability to recite the sutra, and had seen that the occasion was indeed an opportunity to become humble again, and turn to the meaning of the sutra. The devil had not wanted that, so he had sought for and found a copy of the sutra to feed the pride of an expert reciter.

The devotee quietly wrapped up the sutra in the silk, bowed to it with deep reverence, and then turned himself to its meaning. He found the sutra coming to life in his own heart.

All Different

A GIRL began inner training under a Zen abbess for whom she had conceived a great reverence. After a period of probation, she was told by a senior disciple that she would now be given instructions on how to meditate.

"I have never done meditation at all," she said anxiously. "These practices will be ones that suit me, won't they?"

"Yes, they will suit you perfectly," she was assured.

She was given the instructions, and told at the same time that it would be better for her not to discuss her practices with anyone else.

She fully intended to follow the advice, but (as often happens) something slipped out, and she was taken aback to learn that all the pupils had been given these same practices at the beginning.

She asked to see the senior, to whom she complained, "I had expected to receive personal instruction suited to my own temperament. I did ask for that, and you told me that I would get it."

"You have done. These practices will suit your temperament."

"But I've been told that they are just standard practises, which everybody gets. We're all different; there can't be a standardized instruction suitable to everyone, because we're all different."

"Everyone says that at the beginning," remarked the senior.

"But here we do not find it so. We find that we're much the same."

"But the fact that everyone says we are different shows that we must be different," argued the pupil, puzzled.

The answer came quietly, "The fact that everyone claims to be different shows that we're all the same."

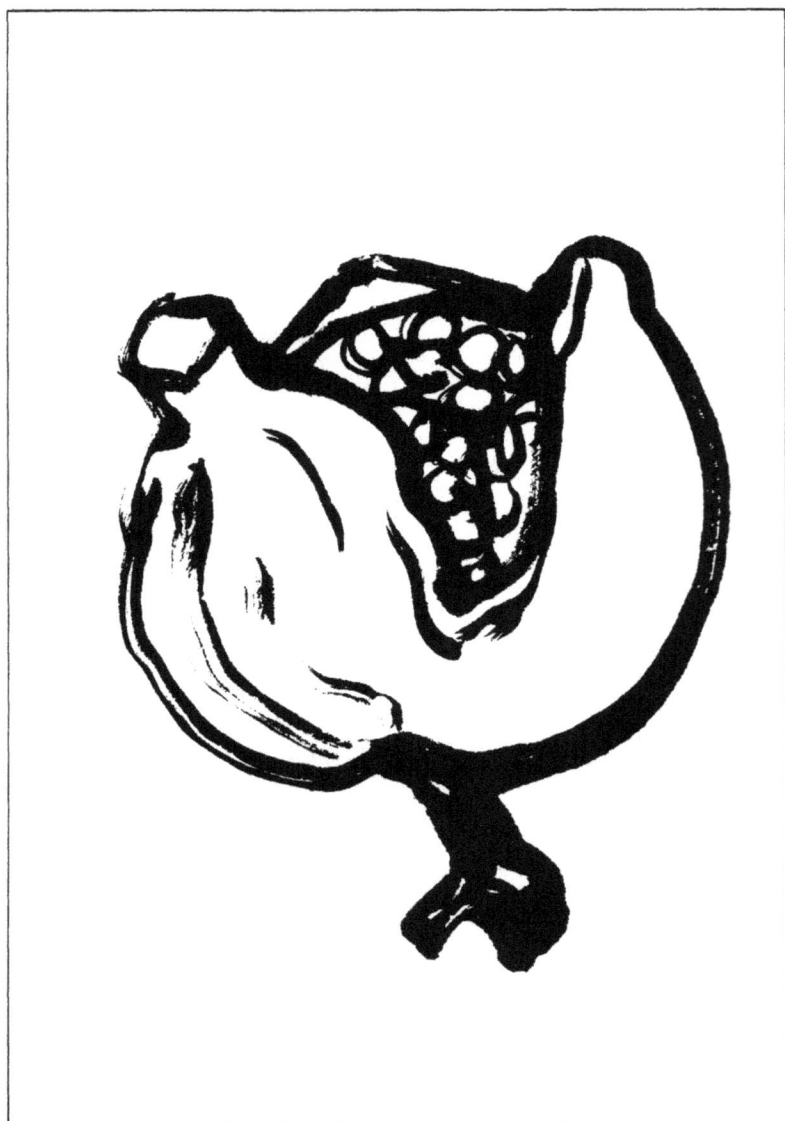

Seeds

NEARLY EVERY sangha from time to time experiences a wave of inertia, which is actively supported by those pupils called the "old soldiers" (and by other less complimentary names). With the aid of various false analogies, propounded with enormous condescension, they try to dissipate all enthusiasm and reduce the whole sangha to their own state of apathy.

On one such occasion, one such person was holding forth to a little group having their morning tea break on a verandah overlooking the garden. He waved a hand at the garden. "Think of the seeds," he said magisterially. "They are sown deep in the ground, and nothing more is seen of them for quite a time. But then the first sprout appears, and a little later the plant or whatever it is. Do you remember when you were very small children, how impatient you used to be, waiting for the seeds to show themselves? You expected something to happen next day or, at most, next week. Some of you may even have dug them up, to see what was happening. How ridiculous it is to the adult, though naturally to the child without experience it seems quite natural.

"Well, it's the same with inner training too. People are far too anxious to see some results, far too anxious. They should understand that once the seeds have been sown, it is a question of waiting, just waiting: impatience for results does nothing to bring them about."

One of the gardeners, an experienced yogi, was passing just below the verandah. "That's right, isn't it now?" the speaker appealed to him for support.

"Yes, that's right. No use expecting seeds to come up the next day, or the next week. But still," he continued, with a negligible glance toward the "old soldier," "if it was ten years ago that you sowed them, and you've never watered the place and you've been walking over it, and then you let a wall collapse on it and didn't clear away the rubble for quite some weeks— well, then, I should think, it might be worth digging them up and sowing some new ones."

Emptying

A TEACHER used to point out to his pupils that what is already full cannot take in any more. This well-known Zen principle is often illustrated by pouring more tea into a filled cup so that it overflows on to the table and floor. This teacher went on to say that when there is a vacuum in the mind, illumination can come to fill it. The pupils did not understand this but let it go, except for one who persistently asked him what he meant exactly. "How can we make a vacuum in the mind?" he would say, to which the teacher made no reply but sat silent.

After some repetitions of this, the teacher told him, "Well, as you are so keen I'll give you some private instruction on it, if you're willing to prepare by purifying yourself," and he gave him elaborate directions for a daily ritual to be continued for three weeks, after which he was to fast for three days.

When all this had been carried out, the candidate came at dawn to the main hall of the temple as arranged, where he found the teacher standing in full robes and looking enormously impressive. The pupil came forward in awe-struck silence, made his salutations, and stood before him. The teacher crashed the end of his staff on to the wooden floor three times, drew himself up to what seemed more than his normal height, and boomed, "I have something very important to tell you. For this, you have purified yourself and fasted. Now attend carefully: such an opportunity is rare."

He paused. The pupil waited for him to continue, but the master merely stood like a statue. The disciple began to think,

"Why doesn't he tell me?" Then he thought, "What on earth is going on?" As the silence lengthened, he realized that such thoughts were useless. He waited. Then he stopped waiting, and just stood still. He began to feel a sort of emptiness spreading out within himself. After a little, in that emptiness he caught a glimpse of a clarity and purity that does not have to speak, does not have to breathe, does not have to think. The teacher broke in abruptly, "The interview is finished. Go away."

In the following months, the emptiness began to return more and more often, bringing with it a kind of coolness and light. Some time afterwards the teacher said to him, "When you are fully expectant for something, and that thing does not come, or comes but is suddenly taken away, there is a vacuum. If you can manage not to fill that vacuum with thoughts of 'Why isn't it here?' or 'Where has it gone?' or 'Why has it turned out like this? What's happening?' then in the emptiness you can have a realization.

"It's the same in worldly life. Suppose you have tried for something and you have worked hard for it, sacrificing yourself for a long time perhaps, even for years, until it has become the whole world to you. Suppose that thing is viciously kicked to pieces in front of your eyes and ceases to exist; it's completely destroyed by mindless spite.

"Now there's a vacuum: Now's the time! If you fill the emptiness with thoughts of resentment and hatred, you'll make no progress from it. But if you can suddenly realize, 'Now I'm free of that, free from it all,' there'll be an emptiness. From emptiness, spiritual inspiration can come to you. If you do that—and you can do it if you try—you will feel a breath from beyond, giving you new life and new wisdom. Those are the times.

"Of course you must practise steadily and hard in the ordinary way, very hard. But great openings come when your whole universe has suddenly collapsed and there's an emptiness."

Silence

A PUPIL asked why they were expected to study the texts. "Surely it is enough if we simply do the practices?"

"Merely to perform the practices, like a pledge fulfilled, will not be effective if there is no inner conviction. The whole personality has to be unified into the practice."

"But why? Can't the disturbing elements of the personality be put down by very strong practice?"

"They may be put down." replied the teacher, "but they may not stay down. A seventeenth-century Japanese Zen master relates how he once met an old priest who talked incessantly, like a waterfall. After a little time, he suggested to the old man that practice of silence was a good thing occasionally.

"Of course it is," shouted the priest. "A very good thing, a very good thing it is, a very good thing indeed. I should know better than anyone, better than anyone. When I was young I practised a vow of complete silence for fifteen years, fifteen full years, I tell you. I never spoke a word during those fifteen years, not a word. I'm the man to tell you about silence," and he proceeded to do so.

Mu in Prison

A JAPANESE businessman saw a cast-iron chance to make a quick profit. He took the capital from a trust fund, meaning to return it almost at once. It happened that a spot-check by auditors revealed what he had done. Though the venture was successful and the money was repaid, it was a serious offense for which he got a sentence of three years' imprisonment. He was sent to a small prison in the north.

He had done a little Zen training some years before, mainly as a means to strengthen his character. During the hardships of prison, he again took up the Mu koan, which he had been given at that time by the teacher.

In an article which he wrote for a magazine, he described how the bad food, cold, and a brutal jailer made him think of suicide, but through the concentration on the Mu he began to feel a sort of metal in himself. After a time he found it recurring to his mind at odd moments during the day. He noticed a patch of small trees and scrub on the snowy mountain slope opposite the prison, which began to look like the compact twelve strokes of the Chinese character for Mu. Sometimes he felt a sensation of inner space, a coolness in the midst of his sufferings.

The day of his release came. He had no fear of disgrace; it was generally recognized that there had been no risk to the money, and though he had broken the law, he had had no intention to swindle, and in fact no one had lost anything. He had just been unlucky.

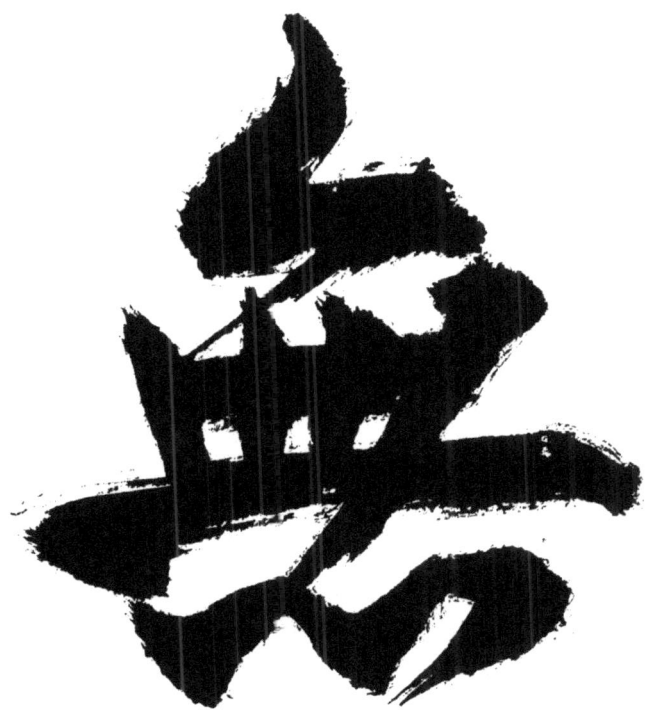

It happened that he was offered an unexpected lift to his hometown and arrived a couple of hours before the family was expecting him. He did not go straight home, because he thought they might be still making preparations for the welcome party which his wife had told him about in her last letter. Instead he walked to a little hill overlooking the house from a distance. It was spring, and when he saw his old home, with the tree in the garden coming into bloom, he burst into tears.

Suddenly he felt in himself the full rush of the great life which interpenetrates the universe. "Why," he cried out, "all is well as it is, as it is. This is the Buddha nature, nothing to be changed, nothing to be changed at all." He felt enlightened.

He had thought of going back to his Zen teacher again, but realized that he did not need any further training now.

Then the thought came to him, "No, I do need it. This apparent enlightenment is based on being back in my hometown, and free. It is no true enlightenment. That little breath of the Mu which I felt in imprisonment—that was genuine, but not this.

"I shall go back to the teacher and train from that."

How Much

A KEEN member of a sangha was always bringing extra furniture for the comfort of the sangha members, and in many other ways trying to make the place and its garden more beautiful and artistic.

A senior member finally dropped a hint that this was not necessary, and was indeed undesirable.

"But I am doing this so that our members should have as nearly perfect conditions for their practice as possible," protested the member. "Surely that can't be wrong?"

"Perfect external conditions are not attainable," said the senior, "and even if they were, external conditions would do little to improve the internal conditions, which is the main point of our training."

"Then are we simply to let the place get dirty and leaky and the garden overgrown?"

"The tradition does not say that," rejoined the other. "There is a minimum necessary, or at any rate, almost necessary. We should be very careful how to pile on so-called necessities beyond that. There is a saying which runs like this:

One bowl of rice and a vegetable each day is necessary;
Two is better;
Three is luxury;
Four makes him ill;
Five kills him."

The Mantra-Sayer

"I ALWAYS recite the mantra of Perfect Realization in the morning, because we are told that recitation of this will infallibly give Nirvana. Then I recite the mantra of Sweeping Away Obstacles in the evening, because we are told that recitation of this will remove them all, and as Realization is something already achieved, the mere removal of the obstacles will reveal it."

"Do you really believe all this?" asked the teacher.

"Yes, I do," replied the mantra-sayer.

"Well, if you really believe in either, you won't need the other one," remarked the teacher. "But you seem to think that each of them could do with a bit of reinforcing."

Notes

"OUR TEACHER," said a disciple to a friend of his, "won't let us take notes when he gives his sermons. Still, he always speaks on one of the classical texts, so as soon as possible afterwards, a group of us meet together and recover as much as we can from memory. With the basic text to consult, we can between us recall nearly everything that he's said, and then we get it down."

"But why won't he allow notes while he's speaking?" asked the friend.

"Yes, we'd always wondered that," went on the disciple. "He just says at the beginning of every year that he doesn't want us to take notes. None of us felt we had the right to ask him; I mean, a teacher's decision mustn't be questioned, must it? But we thought we'd like to know.

"Well, one day when we knew that some outsiders would be coming, we got a notebook and pencil ready. When we saw one keen-looking fellow going in, we just gave them to him. We didn't say anything (the teacher wouldn't have liked that), but we assumed that he'd probably make a note or two.

"And so he did. Soon after the sermon began, he jotted down something. The sermon stopped at once. And then he gave some wonderful teaching." The disciple half-shut his eyes, and continued in a slightly singsong voice:

I don't wish notes to be taken of these talks. It is no use doing it. Some of you may feel that you can take away something in note form, and look over it later on at home, and perhaps then get some sort of enlightenment. But that's a wrong idea. If you are going to get enlightenment, get it here and now, not afterwards. It's the same thing as going to a restaurant where you like the cooking, and instead of eating the food then and there, you wrap it up carefully and take it home with you. Then after some time, maybe next day or next week, you take it out and warm it up in the oven, and expect it to taste good and nourish you. But of course it's no good to you at all.

And then you begin to blame the food, and perhaps the cook as well. The place to eat the food, to take it into yourself and digest it, is when the cook serves it to you. So don't write down notes here, but give full attention to what is said, and take it into your heart.

"Those were his exact words. Isn't it a wonderful teaching, like I said?"

"Yes," said the friend, "it certainly is. But how can you be so sure those were his exact words? It's quite long, and I don't see how you can be sure you remember them perfectly."

"Why, I learned them by heart. We all did. It's wonderful teaching, and we knew it would never be repeated, so we learned it by heart from the script."

"'Script'?" wondered the friend. "What script?"

"Oh yes," confided the pupil. "Didn't you guess? When we gave that visitor the pencil and notebook, so that the teacher would tell him why notes shouldn't be taken, of course there was one of us behind a pillar, taking down what he'd say. We felt that the teaching mustn't be lost."

Faith

A CITY dweller, a keen Buddhist, had to make a business visit to the deep country, and as there was no late train back, he stopped over for one night. In the evening he went to a small temple belonging to a devotional sect. On his return to the city, he described to his teacher what a great effect the service had had on him.

"Those people there, sitting so devoutly and listening intently to the resonant voice of the priest reciting their devotional texts—wonderful! His voice was like a great bell, proclaiming the Buddha to the whole world. I was thinking to myself all the time: how different from the wavering minds and hidden scepticisms of us city folk. One could feel their absolute faith: no lurking doubts there at all."

"No," remarked the teacher. "The only one who might have his doubts would be the priest himself."

The Part

AN EMOTIONAL man was protesting against the principle of Detachment taught in many of the schools of inner training. "It seems to me that this is a negation of all human feeling," he burst out. "Surely when there is an occasion for grief, I should express that grief fully, and when it is an occasion for happiness, I should express that happiness fully, laughing and singing and dancing if I feel like it. And then there are cases where I see something is wrong; I must show that I am against that, absolutely against it."

"Oh, the training doesn't say that sometimes there are not genuine parts to be played. Often there is a genuine role, as you say. But a first-rate actor will manage to express it fully, with the greatest economy of means. Why ham it?"

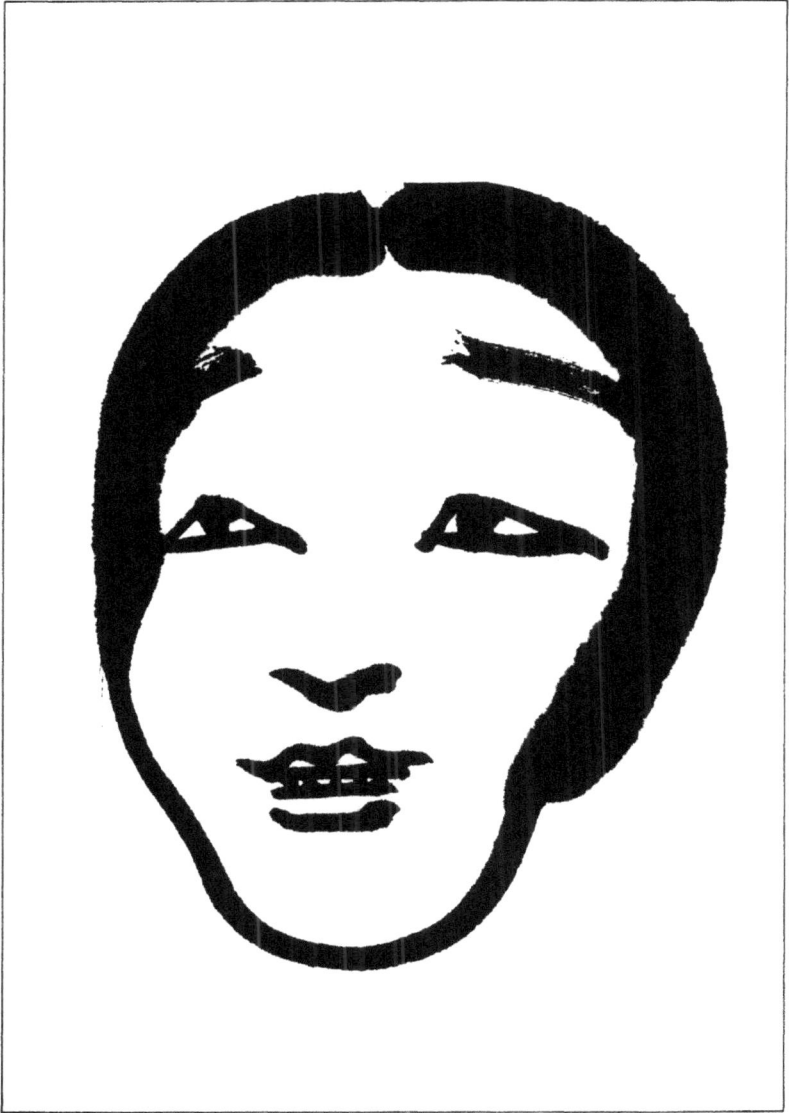

Hero

"SOME OF these youngsters take you as a hero," remarked a friend to a well-known Judo teacher. "Do you think that's a good thing?"

"Well," replied the teacher absently, "it's true that they see what they think are good points, and try to imitate them. But from time to time I give them a hint about where I feel I have made mistakes in life, and how and why it went wrong. I think some of them take it in.

"If they can imitate my good points, and avoid some of my bad ones, then they'll do better in life than I've done. And that'll be some small gain for the world in the next generation, won't it?"

Jobs

A WOMAN disciple who took it upon herself to see that everything in the meditation centre was spotlessly clean and in perfect order, once complained about the slackness of the others. "Some of them," she said to a senior, "just sit there—meditating, I suppose they are—while I am putting things in order. They get there before the meeting, but do they help me put the things out? Oh no, they just get straight on with their meditation. I'd like to just sit there too, like them, but I can't, I'm too busy. The things have got to be put out in the traditional way, and away afterwards, haven't they? But it's always left to me, somehow ..."

After a bit of this, the senior said, "Well, then we'll try something else for a couple of weeks. Now, I've got a bit out of practice at putting the things out and perhaps it would be a good example to others to see me doing it. For the next two weeks, then, you get there early and sit in meditation and you have nothing whatever to do with arranging the meeting."

So the senior was arranging the things while the member sat still, trying to prevent herself from giving reproachful glances at the others sitting alongside her. The arrangements were very simple: There was supposed to be a light in the centre. It had become a sort of tradition that this was represented by three little lights, put on a cloth on the floor in front of the meditators. They were always perfectly aligned at equal distances. There was no rule about where they should be placed, though the arranger generally had placed them exactly in the centre of the cloth. This had come to be expected. About the third day, however, the senior placed the little line just in front of the now meditating member.

As the meeting began, she opened her eyes, and saw with a little start not only the unusual position of the lights (Wrong! said a little voice in her head), but also that they were not quite in line, and that the intervals between them were not the same. She tried to think that she was not concerned with that now, that the senior had done it and doubtless had some good reason. Perhaps, after all, it did not matter. What did it matter? Not at all. Perhaps that was what the senior was teaching. She tried to accept it. But still, something grated. Why change what everyone agreed was a charming and artistic tradition? Next day it was the same. She began to feel an impulse just to put out her hand and adjust the out-of-line light. Just one little touch would do it. But she had been told it was nothing to do with her now. Her body began to fidget slightly. Well, when she got the job back in ten days, she would see it was done right again.

It was a long ten days. At the end she saw the senior again, who said, "It's not necessarily so easy to sit there, is it? We all have this sort of thing, you know. The learned ones who study so hard sometimes think they'd like to have a rest from it, and be like the lazy ones who never open a book. That's what they think. And some of those who've been directed to meditate so hard think how easy it would be just to potter about arranging a few lights and sweeping the floor. Now, what do you want to do?"

The member said, "I understand now a little bit. You tell me what would be good that I should do and let me try and do that."

"Ah," said the senior.

Good

A DEVOUT widow, a woman of clear sight and organizing ability, was the guiding hand behind a great work of charity, which substantially benefited the condition of the poor people of the town. She did this in strict anonymity, but by an extraordinary chance the identity of the secret benefactor leaked out. She began to be respected and even revered by the townspeople.

She remarked to a friend from another town, "I am going to leave this place. I am too highly esteemed here; all this fame and attention interfere with my spiritual practices."

"You need not move," her friend replied. "Quite soon you'll find that envious people are circulating damaging rumors about you. They'll say ... oh, I don't know what it will be, perhaps that you have somehow made something for yourself out of the funds. That's the sort of thing. Then you'll drop into obscurity again, and get your freedom back."

Some months later they met again. "You were right, and I am free once more," said the widow and smiled.

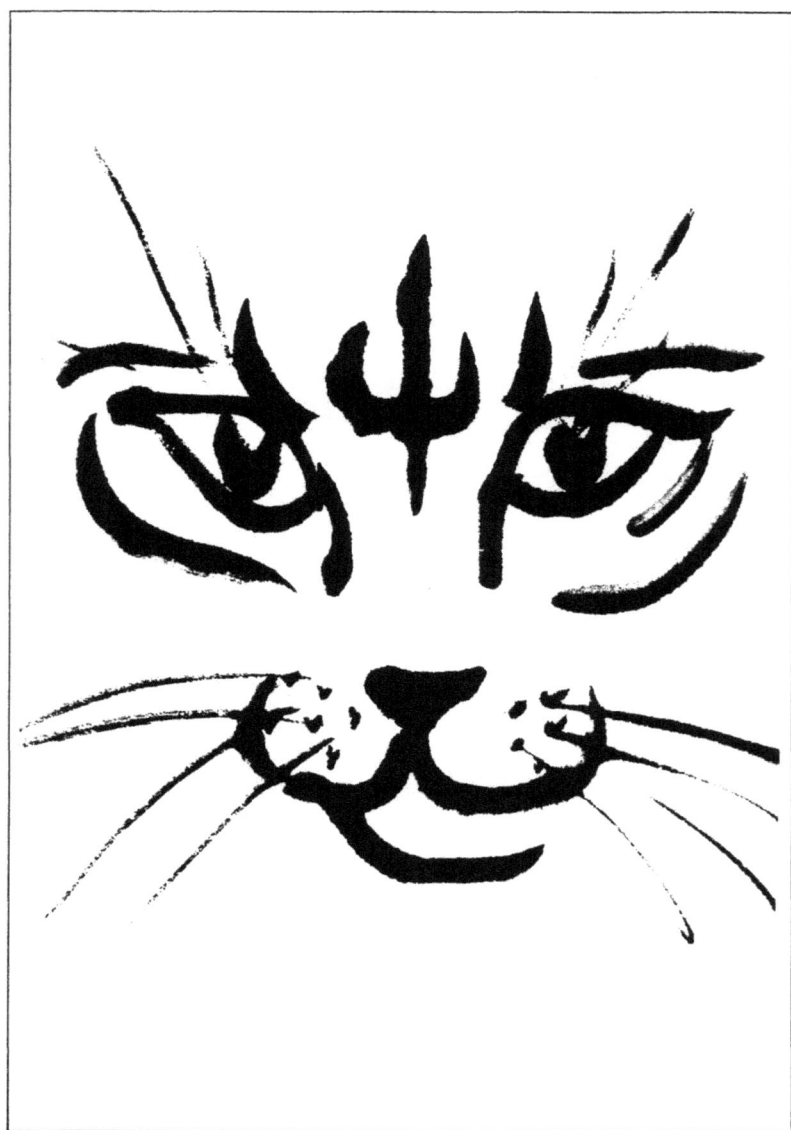

Cat and Dog

IN SOJIJI temple, near Tokyo, there is a picture of the Chinese Zen patriarch Nansen killing a cat. It illustrates a famous koan riddle. With his right hand he is holding aloft the glaring spitting cat, while his other hand grasps the sword. The Japanese master Dogen, founder of the Soto Zen line of which Sojiji is a head temple, remarked of the story, "Buddhism can be taught in this way, but it is open to abuse and best avoided."

A great Indian teacher who saw the picture remarked that the cat represents the mind. One of his pupils was asked about it, and commented:

> The teacher did not care for the company of cats. In the tradition, the cat was the only animal which did not come to mourn the passing away of the Buddha. Devoted to comfort as they are, they teach no spiritual lesson, whereas the dog, intelligent and self-sacrificing, has a lesson to teach.
>
> The dog looks at you and his look says, "How wonderful you are! How I love you! What can I do to serve you?" The cat looks at you and the look says, "How wonderful I am! How you love me! What are you going to do to serve me?"
>
> The untrained mind is a cat, very selfish, but often loved and served by the individual self. It must become a dog, loyal and self-sacrificing, recognizing the superiority of the true human self. Then it becomes not only happier but more intelligent, like the dog, who, recognizing the superiority of the human, is not merely happier than the cat but far more intelligent.

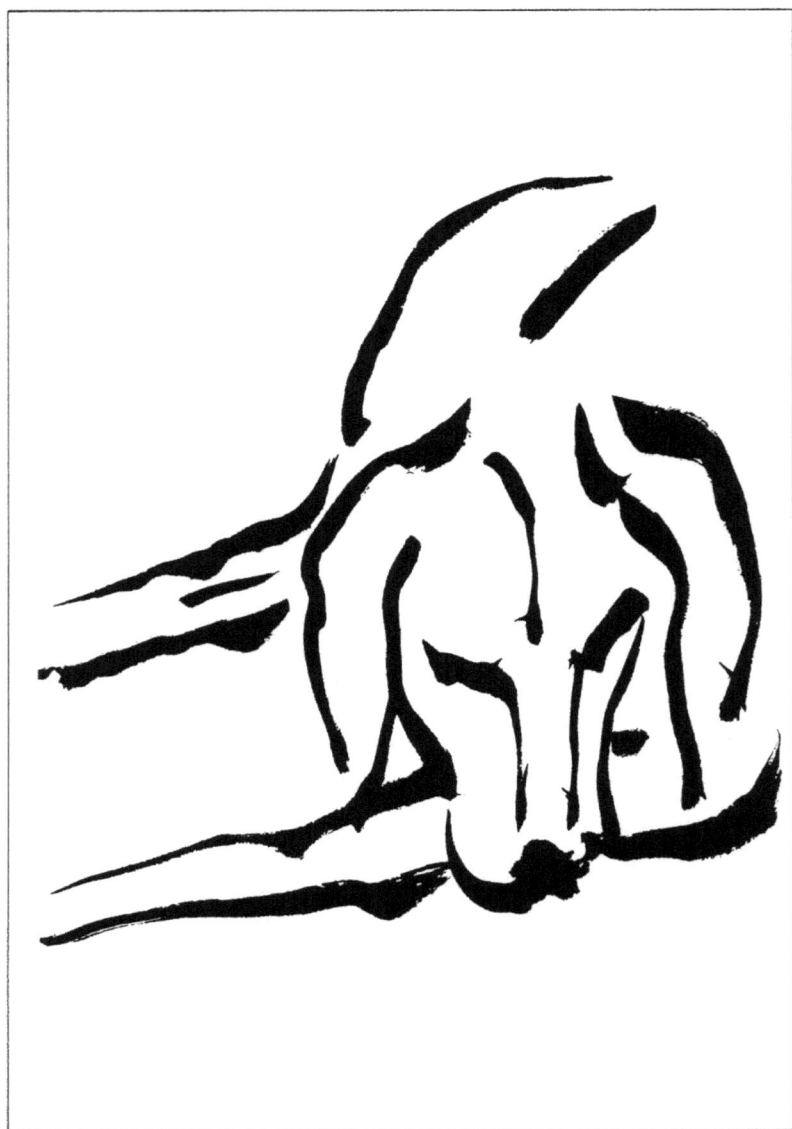

Shooting Arrows

A MONSTER bird, though it did not do much actual harm, terrorized the whole district by its frightening appearance. So a great warrior was asked if he could make it go away or kill it. I have seen a picture of the bird—it is sort of human with a bird's head and wings, and it has a terrifying aspect. The warrior went and started shooting arrows at it, but his arrows did not pierce its body, they stuck to it. So the warrior took his lance and ran at it, but the lance, too, was deflected and just stuck on the bird's body. Then he heaved at it with his sword, but the sword somehow did not make contact but also just stuck. Being a warrior, he also knew of the Jujitsu means as they were then and he tried them, but his hands now also stuck to the bird's body and he was rendered helpless. And the bird-head said, "Now do you surrender?" When he said "No!", the bird was transformed—we need not go into it but it was the God of the Martial Arts and he said, "You have tried with everything you knew, with arrow, lance, sword, and your techniques; all these failed until there was nothing left. You were naked. Nothing, but still ..."

Now this story was taken up by a Zen teacher. When we approach something like Zen (though it is not restricted to Zen) we first of all try shooting the arrows of our opinion, or of information which we have, or of guesses or inference—we try from a safe distance; shooting arrows as we try to pierce it and to find out what it is. But the arrow flies with alien feathers—the feathers in an arrow are not its own, they have come from somewhere else. And further, an arrow may pierce its target but then it is taken out and perhaps used again; the arrow never gets anything. But the bird which flies with its own feathers, when it has made its flight, finds a nest and a mate and has young ones. Moreover, the arrows of opinion will not pierce the target, they will just stick, so will the lance, the sword, and finally the technique until you have nothing left. You have to approach this finality. It is not wrong to try these means, but in the end there has to be nothing left but you. And if you are still determined and not daunted by the failures, then there will be a transformation.

Trick

IN THE 1950s, a stipendiary magistrate of unimpressive build called at the Budokwai Judo Club. I'll call him Henry Symonds. His work took him sometimes into dangerous places where he might be attacked, and he wanted to learn some self-defense. We did not normally teach self-defense to anyone who had not done at least two years' Judo, and could not control their temper. Furthermore, the tricks will not work without precision and balance acquired by considerable training.

He was referred to me, and I explained this to him. He asked, "Is there nothing then?" and I told him that if he joined the Club, and was willing to practise fifteen minutes a day at home, I could show him something. (Our principle was to make the wealthy pay for the poor: some of the keenest young members had very little money.) I told him it would be very boring, but there was something determined about him.

I explained that he would learn only one trick. I gave him three lessons on this very unusual technique: it has the advantage of infallibly surprising an attacker, but the slightest hesitation or imprecision ruins it. He had to build up his practice to 150 repetitions of this each morning; as he mastered it, he could do it in ten minutes. I saw him occasionally for the first few months; when he had mastered it he thought of dropping the practice, but I warned him. "Never miss even one day, however off-colour you may feel. It has to become natural." I suddenly shot a hand toward his eyes, and as he blinked, said, "It's got to become as unconsciously done as that blink."

I heard no more till about thirty years later, after I had retired from Judo and never went near the Judo clubs. Then a young Judo enthusiast came to see me about something quite different. He was a bit in awe of my Judo grade, and seemed slightly embarrassed as he said on leaving, "My uncle is Henry Symonds, and when he heard I had taken up Judo, he gave a message for me to pass to Mr. Leggett, if I ever saw you. He didn't explain it, and I don't know what it means, but anyway I'd like to pass it on now. It's in two words: 'IT WORKED.'"

Gardens

WESTERN MEMBERS of an Eastern sangha were discussing what they agreed was a common difficulty: when a new practice is received solemnly from the teacher there is a feeling of exaltation, but that feeling gradually gets less. It can be revived temporarily by reliving in memory the occasion when this practice was conferred, but these revivals become less and less effective. Finally the practice is liable to become completely dry, pursued only in a dogged spirit of Keep On Keeping On.

As they realized how general the experience was, they decided to ask one of them to put it to the teacher on behalf of all.

When he heard what the delegate had to say, however, he insisted that they should all come together as a group to put their question. After questioning a number of them, and hearing their replies on very much the same lines, namely of wearing off of the spiritual elevation felt at the beginning, in spite of sincere efforts to preserve it, he made a formal reply:

"I asked you all to come here and submit to being questioned to confirm that you were all really concerned with this, and not simply subscribing to something dreamed up by one person.

"You all seem to assume the practices are given to you in order to produce a state of exaltation. But that is not the case at all. A state of exaltation can arise from temporary gratification of an ambition, for instance. There are such higher states of exaltation which arise from the purification of the mind instrument. But none of these things is the purpose of the practices in

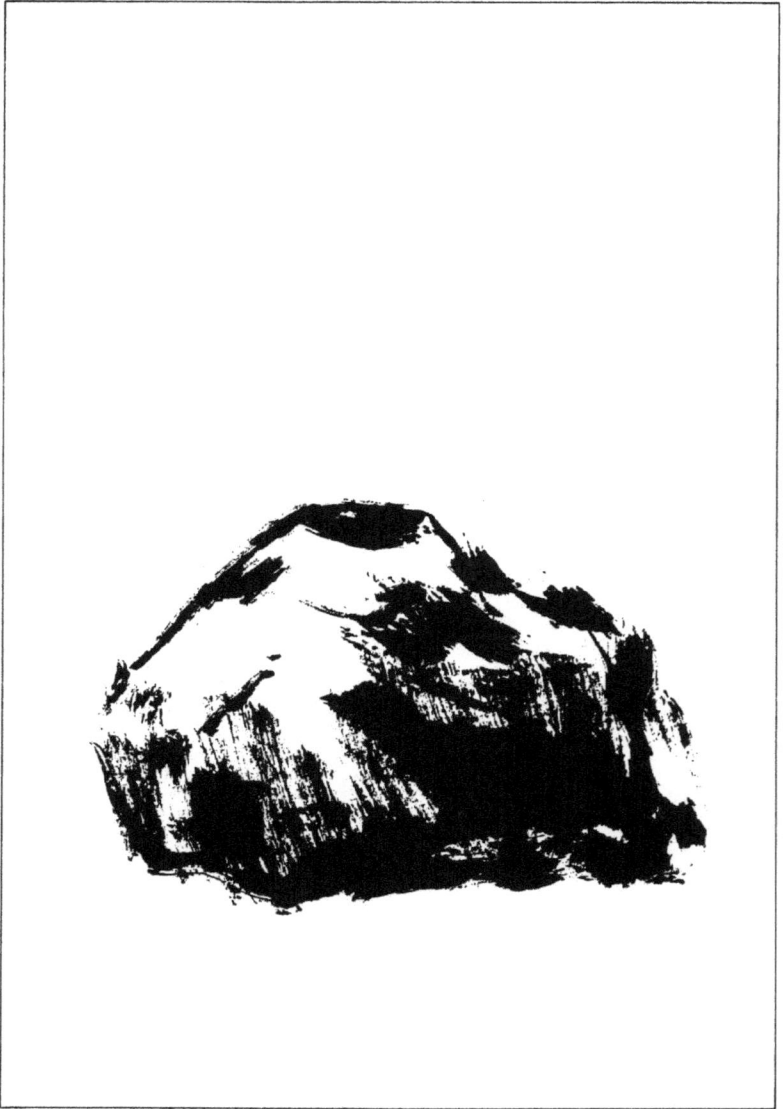

any true tradition. Sometimes, young aspirants, after completing a severe course of training, or making a great renunciation, seem to shine like torches. But it goes off after a time.

"There seems to be a Western tendency to think in terms of negative or positive exclusively, triumph or disaster. I have heard that in your Bible you have a book of Jubilees, but there is also a book of Lamentations. The two go together.

"When we look at pictures of your famous gardens, we see the same thing. They depend on large expanses with many flowers: in the summer they are ablaze with colour, but in the winter they look deserted and melancholy. At one time they are glad; at the other season, they are sad. The two go together.

"But the famous gardens in Japan do not depend on passing things like flowers. There may be some flowers, but the garden does not depend on them for its effect. The rock gardens, for instance, may consist of little more than rocks and carefully raked sand. To a Western eye, I am told, there seems to be nothing much there at first glance. But after a time, the proportions of the garden begin to have an effect on a silent onlooker. He begins to feel that there is a peace in the garden, and soon afterwards he feels a peace in himself. After a fall of snow, the proportions of the garden are still able to convey that peace: snow can even add to the beauty of the garden.

"The general tradition in the East has been to aim at freedom from the alternation of bad and good, negative and positive, sad and glad. The goal is peace. You have this tradition in Christianity also—the peace that is beyond understanding. But it does not seem to be given the central place.

"When you take up a practice here, disregard feelings of exaltation or depression; for a long time these will come and go across the surface of your mind. But go deeper than the surface: by your practice penetrate to the very depths of the mind, and finally beyond even that. Then you will find peace, and freedom from all passing alternations."

Independence

1. THERE WAS a Zen class attended by many foreigners that I had heard about when I was in Tokyo. The teacher carried a stick and said, "If you do not sit properly, I will hit you with this stick." Then he shouted, "Don't raise your shoulders like that, drop your shoulders. I shall walk slowly and watch you, but don't be nervous, drop your shoulders, and if I see you sitting calmly with shoulders dropped, I won't hit you at all. Or maybe I'll hit you twice as hard!" You have to consign yourself to your teacher. There has to be complete resolution to go through anything.

2. A VERY poor Brahmin poet composed some verses for a Moslem ruler who, most impressed, ordered a great pile of silver coins to be given as reward. The Brahmin refused to accept the silver unless the gift was made in the traditional fashion, that is, the giver must bow when the gift is bestowed. This the Moslem refused to do. "Think well," said the ruler, pointing to the silver, "where will you find a patron like this?"

"And where will you find an independent man like this?" said the Brahmin, kicking over the pile of silver as he walked out.

We are not asked to do things like this very often, but we have to be ready to do something like it sometime in our lives. We have to do it not whiningly and grudgingly, but with a kick of independence as we walk away.

Gone Away

IN SOME Japanese temples, there are glass cases in which are displayed ancient manuscripts, relics of the founder, and so on. There are no professional guides, and young monks learn the information by heart, stand beside the case, and recite it. I remember in one temple the guide stood upright beside the case, saying his piece without himself looking at the exhibit. At one point we moved on to a certain case from which the exhibit had been removed, for cleaning or some research. The monk did not notice, but gave his description in a firm voice: "Here is …" Only after about a minute did he notice that we were not looking at the case, and himself peered into it. "Oh," he said, "oh, it's gone away …" and led us on to the next.

I was reminded of this when I heard a teacher say how many of the temples in China early in this century had been still magnificent, but "the gods had departed." The majesty of the buildings, and the splendour of the services, and the sonorous syllables of the holy texts were saying, "Here is the truth; come and worship." But the thing they were describing had gone away.

Ghosts

A MERCHANT who lived near a graveyard got the idea that ghosts from the graves were threatening to enter his house. He got a spell from a priest and went over the graveyard at sunset as he had been told, reciting the spell with all his force. "You have to feel that you are spitting out all your insides with the spell," the priest had instructed him. At first he was trembling with fear, but after a little he felt the effects of the spell, and finally realized that the ghosts had been quelled.

He boasted of his success to a friend, a man who had attained discernment through Zen practice. "You don't have anything like this in your Zen, I suppose."

"I wouldn't say there's nothing like it," replied the friend, "but in Zen the question would have to be asked, what is this being done for? And what about the feelings of the ghosts? They may have been subdued, but they are still there, aren't they? Surely this is not the right way."

"Then what ought I to do?" asked the merchant.

"Get another prayer, this time for the salvation of ghosts. They will become freed from the bonds of unfulfilled karma which still hold them here, and there will be no more ghosts. That is the right way to meet ghosts, inner and outer."

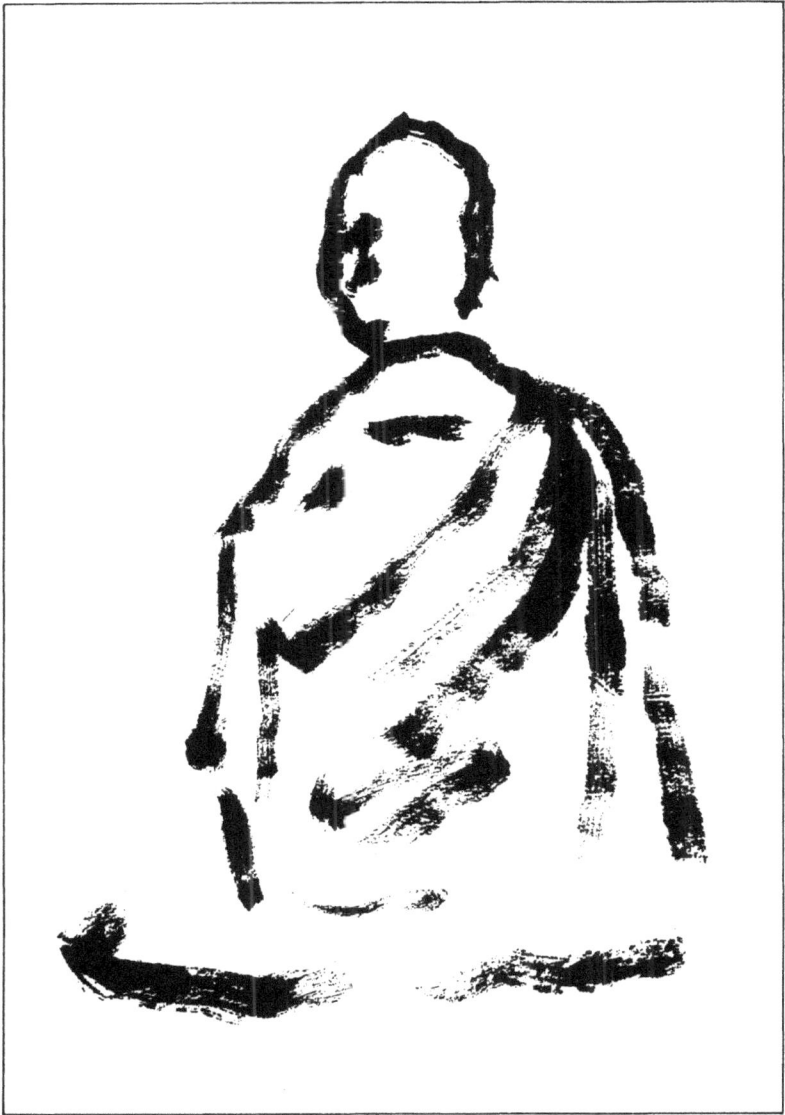

The Pond

IN ONE of the oldest Japanese temples, there is a small pond. It is irregular in shape, but admired by visitors—especially foreign visitors—for the subtle aesthetic effect of the design.

At the end of one such enthusiastic foreign visit, the head monk remarked confidentially in Japanese to a foreigner whom he knew well, "This pond is not old, though it has been allowed to become old-looking. As a young monk, I was one of those who dug it. Six of us began together in the middle of the space, and we simply dug outward from the centre. Of course, the stronger monks got further out than the weaker ones. After a few days, the old head monk came to see it. He said, 'Stop! Now bank up the sides with the big stones, and leave it. See that the moss is allowed to grow over the stones.'

"As I look at it now, I do find it attractive. But when it's so admired, I feel tempted to tell them how it got made, and ask them this: Who should get the credit for the design: the strong monks, the weak monks, the old head monk, or something else?"

Fallacy Somewhere

A BUDDHIST was trying to point out to a sceptic the superiority of Buddhism, as suitable for a rational person. "In religions, there is always a dogma, which has to be believed or at least subscribed to. In Buddhism there is no such requirement. The Buddha simply presented his view and asked listeners to apply their own reason: if it seemed reasonable to them, they should adopt it."

The sceptic produced an unexpected rejoinder. "As a matter of fact, the Buddhist presentation contains a fallacy which religions in general do not suffer from. The fallacy is this: the Buddha's conclusion was that the mind of the ordinary man is stained and swayed by passion and delusion, and therefore incapable of seeing the truth. So far, it is undeniably the fact. In Buddhist practice, there is a long process of purifying the mind before truth is realized. And yet, there is the Buddha telling people who have never done the practice to use their reason to judge his doctrine! On his own showing, that unpurified reason will be unable to judge between truth and falsehood. It will give him a doubtful report every time. That's why it would be more reasonable to believe dogmas, which at least claim to come from a divine source of truth.

"Your Buddhism is like handing a camel-hair brush to someone whose eyes are full of grit, and telling him to use it to get the grit out. The eye itself, which is necessary to the operation, is the very thing which is impaired. The only reasonable thing for such a patient, nearly blind himself, is to find someone else to get his eyes clean. It is the same with perception of ultimate truth: surely you see that?"

The Buddhist was bewildered and did not know what to say. That evening he asked his teacher, who said, "I have told you in the past not to argue with combative sceptics. Such debates are fruitless and do not lead to truth; they go on endlessly."

"But it seems to me that this point *was* reasonable, as he said it was. Surely we need to know how to meet this sort of doubt?"

"It can be met, but to meet it gives no spiritual satisfaction; it is simply a matter of words. For instance, he was admitting the uncertainty of reason in order to attack the Buddha.

"The Buddha used to point out that his own conclusions could be confirmed by anyone through practice. The real test is experience. And as a matter of fact true religions all say the same thing: their statements are not meant to be mere dogmas blindly or fanatically accepted. I've seen in the Upanishad called Brihadaranyaka, which is much older than the Buddha's time, how first an ancient sage's experience of truth is described. He was already long before 600 BC. Then it adds, 'And to this day, it is the same for whoever knows, in like manner.' Over a thousand years after that, the great philosopher-yogi of India confirmed, 'On this point, there is no difference between the spiritual giants of the past and the little people of today.'

"All can realize truth in the same way. But truth is not weakened, or strengthened, by clever debating points."

Dark Spotlight

IN ONE of the weekly discourses to a small group of disciples from the country, the subject of egoism was raised on several successive occasions. The speaker remarked that people who had done a little training were of course aware that they ought not to perform their good deeds to the sound of trumpets, as it were. "But," he added, "there is a way of coughing when putting a gold coin in the collection bowl, which is really the same thing. Let our motto for a few weeks be: 'No coughing when practising virtue.'"

As they left to return to the country, one woman disciple confided to her friend, "I cannot understand why when we are there the teacher keeps on talking about egoism as a great barrier."

"Perhaps he thinks we are egoistic," replied the other. "I always try to examine my conduct afterwards and usually find something on those lines."

"You can speak for yourself of course—I have nothing to say about that. But me—how could anyone think me egoistic? I always keep in the background. I do all that service without any attempt at getting recognition for it. Why, I'm *famous* for my love of obscurity!"

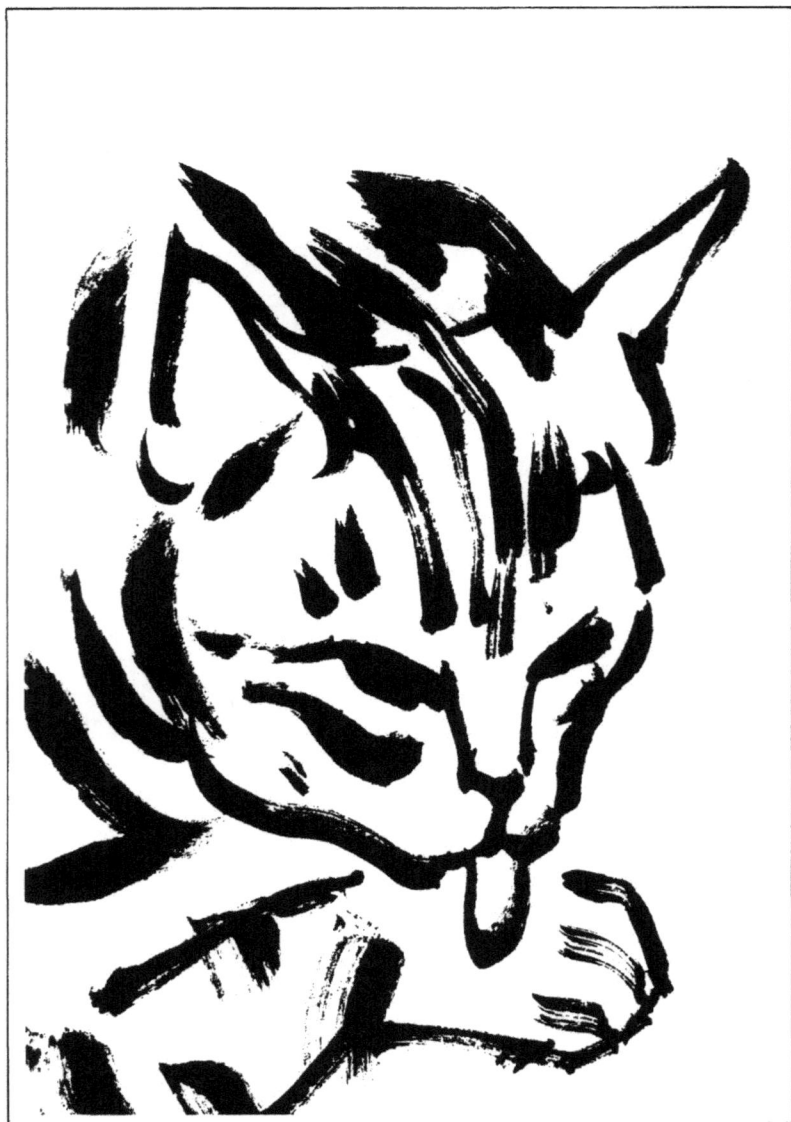

Cleaning

A ZEN teacher was asked to visit a hippie community, and when he arrived they were lined up to meet him.

He said afterwards, "All the men had one leg of their frayed trousers shorter than the other; the women's clothes were ill-fitting and not too clean. Both sexes had their hair in a tangle."

In a Zen monastery, however poor the clothes may be, they are always clean, and carefully adjusted.

After the talk and meditation session, one of the community said in a puzzled tone, "Why do Zen followers lay such stress on tidiness? Surely it's an obsessive concern with trivialities. What do such things matter? They don't have anything to do with the big things of life. To be always fussing about them is just a burden on the mind."

The teacher saw the community cat passing, and snapped his fingers. The cat came up and the teacher gave it a little milk. The cat purred, sat down, and began to clean itself vigorously.

"He likes doing that," remarked the teacher. "Cleanliness and desire for beauty are among the deepest instincts."

"But for men," argued the other, "surely we should be concerned with what's really important, not with such artificialities. Surely it's not right to spend much time and energy on artificial tidying?"

"One can be artificially untidy too," replied the teacher. "It's a sort of defiance, and has nothing to do with what's really important."

Spitting

IN A traditional-style Japanese home, or a temple today, the floor consists of straw mats, beautifully constructed with exact precision. Life is lived on the floor, the whole building being raised a couple of feet off the ground. The mats and the wooden corridors are kept spotlessly clean, and no dirt from outside is allowed to enter; shoes are left in the porch located on the ground level.

The avoidance of what is called *aka,* which can be roughly translated as dirt, grime, or anything greasy or slimy, has always been a major preoccupation in Japan. For instance, in the first half of this century, a Japanese girl would tend to hesitate on entering a Western-style classroom at school. Her instinct was to remove her shoes, so as not to bring the dirt of the playground into the classroom.

Again, Japanese women wear with traditional dress a pair of white cotton socks. An aristocratic Kyoto lady on her "at home" day used to change her socks when one visitor left, before receiving the next one. Socks that had been worn for even an hour were, so to speak, notionally impure.

In some countries of East Asia, however, at the beginning of this century, the village dwellings had a floor of earth, and life was lived on rough chairs and tables. As in Western life, dogs could freely enter a house if they belonged to the home. In such villages, some of the men had a habit of chewing betel-nut leaves, and spitting out the remaining fibers. It makes a brilliant red splotch on the ground, but is soon trodden in when outside the home. There were some who did not bother to make any distinction between the inside and outside of the house.

A Buddhist from such a village came to train at a temple in Japan. He was very keen and had made some progress in the language before coming, which is rather rare in foreign visitors, and accordingly impressed his hosts. Looking round the temple, he at once realized that his almost unconscious habit of spitting on the floor would be quite inappropriate in these spotless surroundings, and he made great efforts to remember not to do so. But occasionally the force of old habit became too strong, and he would pass on his way unaware that he had left a red splotch in a corner of the room. The first few times it happened it was pointed out to him, with increasing resentment by the monks, and he always apologized profusely and hastened to clean it up. But he still had lapses.

After one such lapse, the head monk was talking about it to the old abbot over tea. He was a perfectionist and expressed his disgust freely.

"Do you think that our new monk is making efforts to get rid of this regrettable habit?" asked the abbot.

"Oh yes, he's very sincere. In a way, he's as distressed by it as anyone. It's not his sincerity that is lacking; it's simply that the culture he comes from can hardly be called a culture at all. It's really a sort of animal life that they're living, judging from this sort of habit."

He noticed that the abbot had absently picked up the tea cloth and was wiping up a few drops of tea and crumbs that had evidently fallen on the floor. He went on, "It seems to me that with such a huge gap between their way of living and ours, it's rather useless for him to come here to train. It's a nuisance for our people to have to go round mopping up these stains whenever they see them."

The abbot was vigorously mopping with his tea cloth at the floor round the table.

"Oh, it's all right here, teacher. He's not allowed in this room. He hasn't been here, spitting on the floor in that disgusting way of his."

The abbot still plied his cloth, and the head monk stopped abruptly. He suddenly realized that there are other, more venomous forms of spitting than the merely physical one.

He changed the subject, and the abbot stopped mopping.

Time, Time

IN JAPAN in the thirteenth century, old people who were deemed useless were taken up a mountain to die. In this case, a son decided his father had to go since he had become a burden. "We are going to take grandpa to the top of the mountain and leave him there," he told his own little son. The boy, who was fond of his grandpa, asked why he couldn't stay at home with them. "No," said the father, "it is kinder that way, when old people are confused and useless." They got a dilapidated sedan chair, bundled the old man into it, and went to the mountaintop. The child asked his father to take grandpa out of the chair and bring it down.

"No, there's no need, this is an old chair, no use to anyone."

"But I need it for you when your time comes," said the boy.

It's nice to record that the father reconsidered and they brought grandpa down.

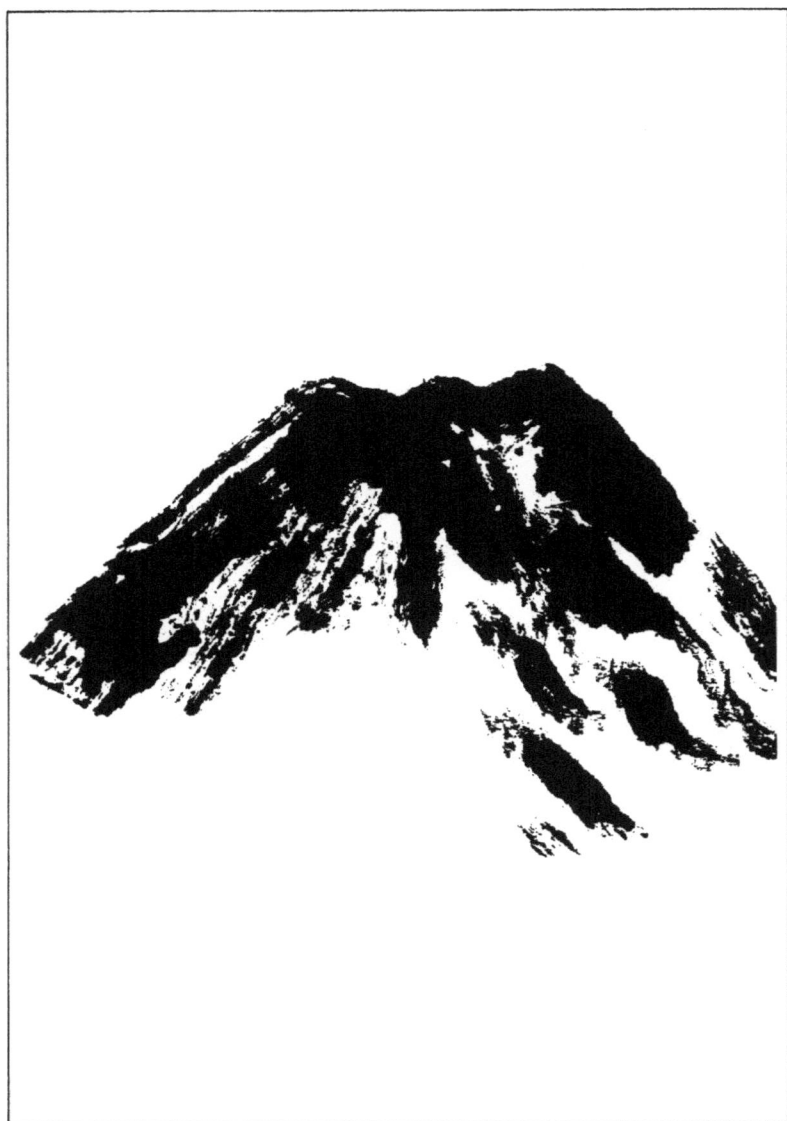

The Blue Mountains

"I DON'T think I want to undertake inner training," remarked a layman to a teacher, "because after all, what guarantee is there that I would be able to bring it to a conclusion? There is no assurance, and it would be a waste of a lot of time and effort if I took it up and then found I couldn't complete it."

"The same applies to any plan which you make," came the answer, "and yet you continue to plan—to move to a better house, to send your children to a good college, and thousands of other things.

"In one tradition, the state of spiritual fulfillment is called the Blue Mountains—where the saint-ascetic lives in contemplation and has the freedom of all worlds. The concluding line of a famous poem runs:

The place he has reached when he dies,
That is his Blue Mountains.

"A true man sets out on the Way and pursues it dauntlessly until he drops. But you have dropped before you set out."

Paid For

IN THE Tang dynasty, a Zen monk was preaching in the open air to a small crowd. A seller of pears, pushing his cart of fruit with its two long handles, paused to listen. He became more and more impatient with the teaching about restraint of passions and inner serenity; finally he shouted, "What can your Buddha do? Show us a miracle if you want us to listen to you!"

"Miracles have to be paid for," replied the monk, "and they bring no lasting good. But practise self-restraint and meditation, and you will be free from sufferings forever."

"Talk, all talk!" retorted the peddler angrily, and he forced his cart through the crowd up to the front. "Your Buddha did miracles, didn't he? Then you do one, if you call yourself a Buddhist."

"The Buddha passed six years in austerities, living on one rice-grain a day. If you did that, you would experience miracles. But he gave them up, and he never taught them to his disciples. He never taught miracles as a way of ending suffering."

"That's a get-out, just a get-out! Show us something, show us something."

The crowd began to take it up. "Yes, he's right. Show us something, show us something."

The monk suspended his teaching. He looked at them impressively. "Clear a little space," he commanded, and then stretched forth his hand.

From the ground sprouted, with breathtaking speed, a pear tree, two of its boughs heavy with fruit. The monk stepped forward and broke them off. He went round, distributing the pears to the people. When they were finished he walked quickly away, and the crowd dispersed.

The seller of pears, his mouth still open with amazement, pulled himself together. He looked round and saw his cart. The two long handles had been broken off and it was empty of pears.

Triumph

A PIECE of advice which can be most useful in life runs something like this:

> Aim at success, never at triumph. If you have aimed at success merely, then whether you meet with that or with failure, you will not be upset. You will not get excited, because your personal feelings have not been bound up with your action. But if you have aimed at triumph, then when it comes off, you will become overelated and want to tell everyone about it; and in failure you will get depressed or perhaps angry. In which case you will find yourself either trying to conceal it, or else blaming it on other people. So aim at success, never at triumph.

I once had an experience which brought this advice to life for me. I was given the job of sweeping the leaves away from one courtyard of a Japanese temple. Such courtyards are often covered with moss, and there are small trees which come into leaf at different times of the year, to give the moss the shade which it needs. Moss is regarded as a symbol of spiritual progress in Japanese Buddhism: its growth cannot be forced, but if all weeds are removed, it does make surprisingly fast progress.

The leaves were falling from the trees in this particular courtyard: some were on the ground and others were very loose. I swept the fallen leaves carefully from the surface of the moss into a heap which I then transferred into the bag provided. I wanted to leave the courtyard absolutely clear of leaves, absolutely. In other words, I wanted a triumph. This was one of the first jobs I had been given in the temple, and I wished it to be done perfectly. But I found that when I had swept the ground clear from under several of the trees, one or two more leaves then fell, marring the unbroken greenness of the moss carpet. With some irritation I walked across, snatched them, and stuffed them into the bag. Then a few more fell on another part which I had already swept.

I found myself becoming annoyed, and then angry. I was fairly strong, and as an experienced Judo man, I knew how to apply strength. So I took hold of each tree in turn and shook it violently. All the leaves which were at all loose came down in a shower. I then swept the whole lot up with powerful strokes of the besom. I felt like a man who had just won a Judo contest, in this case, however, against trees. I triumphantly surveyed the courtyard, now absolutely clear of leaves.

As I turned to go, with the full bag, I noticed a monk watching me. He said something to the effect that this was perhaps a little brutal, was it not? "We just sweep up every day the leaves that have fallen. If some more come down where we have already swept, we will sweep them up tomorrow."

Years later, I read something by Mamiya, a great Zen master and poet of the early twentieth century, about sweeping leaves. From my own experience of annoyance at the trees, I could understand his meaning. I felt that perhaps he had had the same experience when young, and that it applied to much more than sweeping courtyards:

We sweep up the leaves that have fallen,
But we do not hate the trees for dropping them.

To the Last Drop

A WOMEN'S charitable organization gradually came to be dominated by an energetic member, skilled in committee procedures and expert at shouting down arguments against her plans. She began to use the meetings as a vehicle for self-display, and for giving expression to her personal likes and dislikes. Quite soon there was a marked deterioration in the organization's activities, but most of the members were afraid to oppose her.

The only one who was courageous enough to do so was the disciple of a Zen teacher. She got no support from her timid fellow members in her attempts to get things back on to a proper basis, and was instead subjected to a campaign of vilification, not stopping at personal physical attacks of a minor nature.

She made no complaint, but the teacher came to hear of it, and one day said to her, "What is your feeling under this persecution?"

She said, "Well, I suppose I try to feel sorry for her because of the bad karma which she is piling up by destroying a benevolent activity."

"No use at all!" cried the teacher. "That sort of attitude is no good, it'll only tire you out, and anyway, you won't be able to keep it up—no one can. Now—think this: YOU'VE GOT TO DRINK DOWN THAT POISONOUS VENOM TO THE VERY LAST DROP. There is a verse:

Set free the bird to fly in the infinite sky of your tolerance;

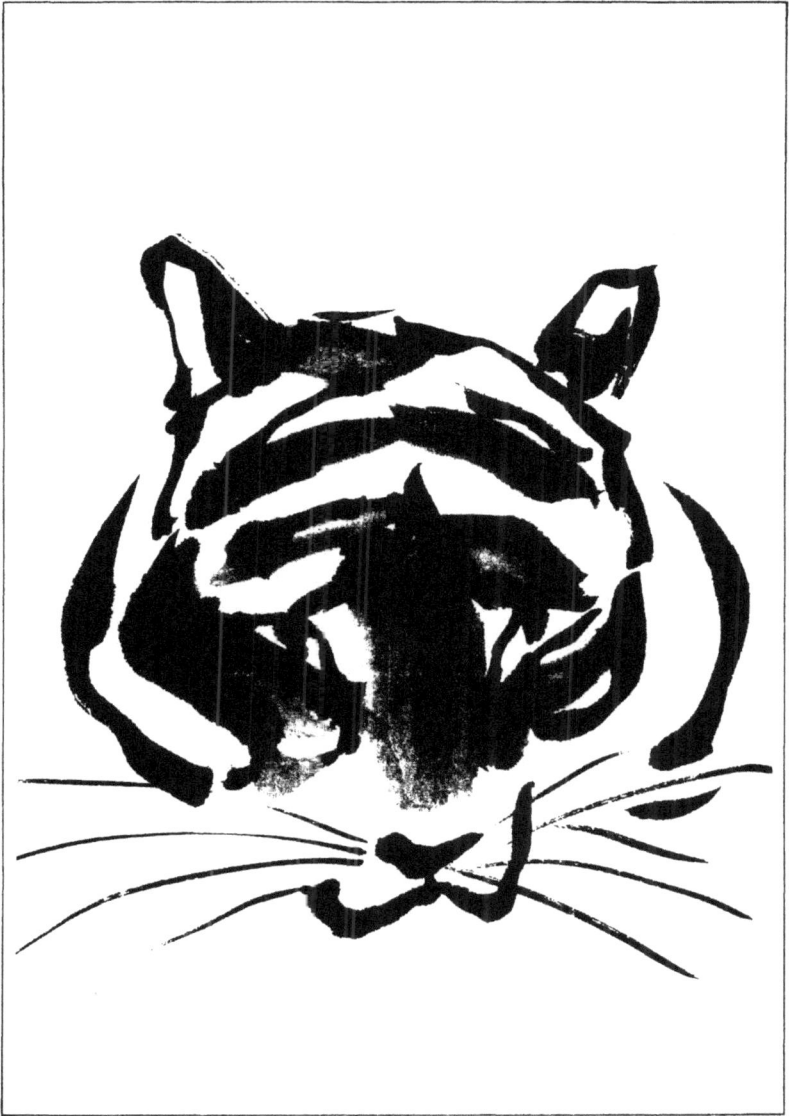

Loose the fish to swim in the boundless ocean of
   your forgiveness.

"Live that."

She said, "But what are we to do? She is not only vicious, but destructive too. Are we simply not to oppose her? I have opposed her and she hates me for it. Are we just to let her have her way, out of love and forgiveness and tolerance? Others are now beginning to join me; people are slowly realizing what is happening."

The teacher looked at her with his eyes wide open. "What you do must come from love. It does not mean doing nothing— the words and acts of love are not always kind on the surface. You may oppose her—in fact you should do so. But it must be for the sake of the benevolent work of your organization, and it must be on a basis of love.

"If you cannot act from love, you may succeed, but you will probably end up just like her. Very likely she herself began as a reformer; having been successful, she got carried away by it. Tiger-slayers often end up as tigers themselves.

"And if you yourself are successful, don't seek triumph; be satisfied with success. Then make it easy for her, if she seeks to shed this role in which she has got caught. Probably she is already sick of it, but cannot get out of it. Let the glacier melt slowly, under the gentle spring sun."

Wisdom Water

A NUMBER of Sanskrit words came into Japanese along with Mahayana Buddhism, one of them being *prajna,* which means transcendental wisdom.

A Japanese politician wrote an article, in the course of which he described how he and two or three others had made a visit to a Buddhist temple to find out whether all was well with the temple lands, and if not, whether they could do anything to help. The abbot received them kindly and the discussion was amiable. There were only a couple of very minor matters, which could easily be set right, and they promised to do them.

The abbot then invited them to lunch, and a vegetarian meal was served, very well cooked. The abbot asked whether they would like anything to drink with it, and the politician took this to be an invitation to have some Japanese rice-wine. He therefore said that he and his companions would welcome a little saké.

To his amazement, the abbot strongly reprimanded him, saying it was a disgrace to utter such a vulgar word in the sacred precincts. The politician knew that many Buddhist priests do in fact permit the use of wine, provided it does not lead to intoxication; he assumed that this temple was a particularly strict one, and he apologized profusely for his suggestion.

The abbot accepted the apologies with a dignified inclination of the head. He called his attendant, and said, "Serve our guests with some Prajna-water." The politician wondered what

Wisdom Water might be, and prepared himself for something on the lines of a fruit-juice drink.

When the Wisdom Water came, however, it turned out to be saké of high quality. It had been only the word that was prohibited, not the thing itself.

Channel

SOME PEOPLE say that although they meditate and do practice, there is no response from the True Face within. A teacher gave this example: "Suppose you are an electrician and are rung up to go round at once for some urgent repair but then come back again complaining that there was no one in. You then telephone the place and are told, 'I have been in all the time waiting for the electrician! Why don't you come?' 'But I rang the bell and rang and rang and there was no answer!'" The teacher said that in the same way repairing the bell is our immediate task when we practise. Then there will be a response.

Theoretically we know that the air is full of radio waves. But people might ask, "Where are these waves?" And we say, "Oh, but they are here." One may want to listen to them, but when one is banging and shouting one cannot hear anything! Or if one has but a little set, even a little banging and shouting, and I cannot hear. This is a delicate analogy. The receiving set is not perfect for a long time but the sound is there. In the same way, the teacher said, we are spitting at the Buddha all day long, and then in the evening we are shouting at the Buddha. But if we reduce the noise, reduce the shouting, reduce the banging, reduce the clamour, "I don't see him!" Then he can be perceived!

A teacher said, "There is all the difference in the world between a man who is inviting the Buddha into his own home but stands in the door so that the Buddha cannot come in, and another who stands aside, becoming nothing, and so the

Buddha can come in." In the same way, standing out in our meditation and daily life practice, we are in the way. Although we are inviting and seeking, we are actually in the way, and the thing is to melt into and become a vacancy through which the Buddha can come. And he said that the practices to this purpose are not very attractive, or they are attractive at first, which is one understanding of the "beginner's mind" and why the beginner's mind is so highly praised. In the beginning we are thinking and pondering about the practice all the time, in our daily life we can hardly wait and exercise patience, or whatever else it might be. We must not forget that urgency because the time will come when we will merely think, "I'll do it, I'll do it, YES, I'll do it." Think back then to the beginner's mind. Usually we start with enthusiasm, then we have a "dead" period when we think it is always going to be like this, always going uphill and somehow dreary and dull. Where then is the joy in this? There is not, really, and what you felt at the beginning was actually no joy but hope. A modern analogy says that it is like that with cigarettes and whisky. Nobody enjoys the first cigarette they smoke, they only smoke them in order to appear more grown-up than they are. And nobody likes the first whisky or other alcohol, rather they spit them out if they can. Yet these two can become the strongest addictions. This may not be a particularly elevating example, but it is a powerful one. In the same way, Zen Buddhist practice can open up and become a joy like no other joy.

Pearls

AT THE end of a talk on Buddhism by a well-known master, a Western listener irritably objected. "You kept saying that while our whole life was a life of distinctions, we should be in illusion and suffer. You quoted all those stories of rich people groaning because they thought themselves very poor, or people standing up to the neck in fresh water and crying out, 'We're thirsty!' All very pathetic. But you contradict yourself, because your words themselves are distinctions. So your very words are part of it all: they are just as illusory as the rest."

"Yes," said the preacher, "they're imitation pearls thrown to people pretending to be beggars. But it makes them feel better, just for a bit. And when they feel better, they might stop groaning and wailing for a moment, and look around at how things really are."

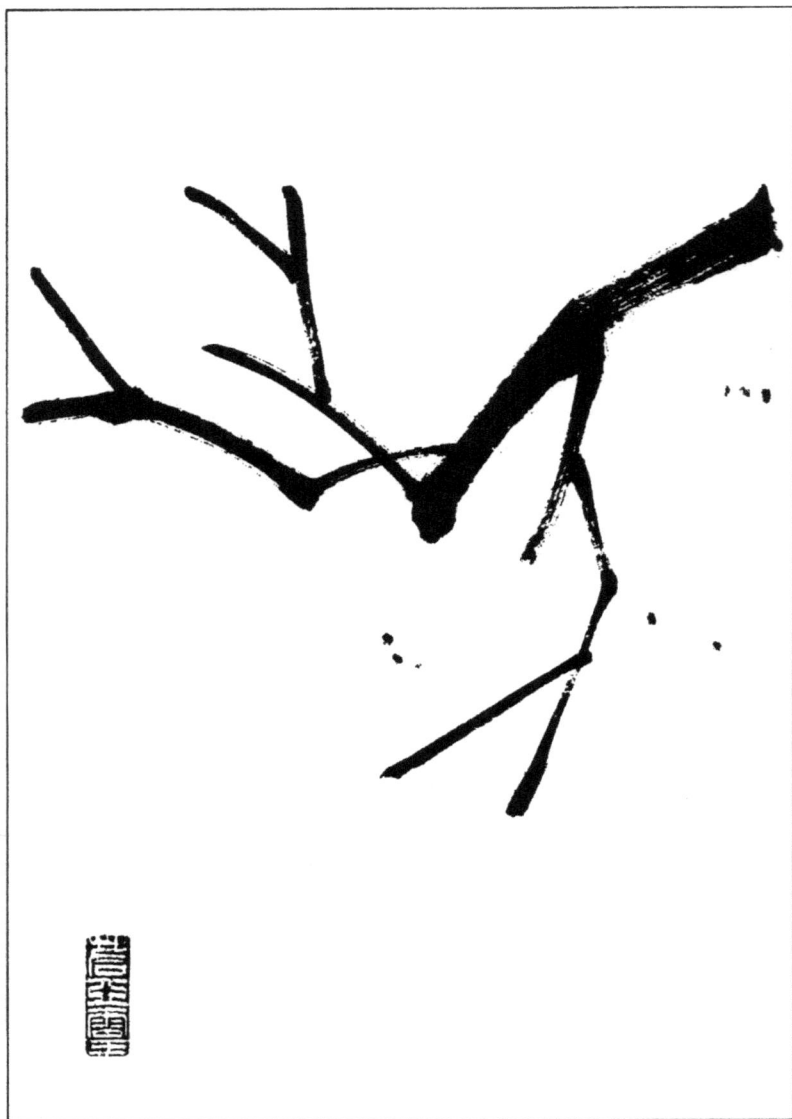

Interlaced Trees

A WOOD of trees growing together can get the branches interlaced so that the trees support each other. Even if the root has become very shallow, the whole thing looks like a stable structure, a sort of table with many legs. But because there are no deep roots, it all collapses helplessly in a storm. A society or group, says a seventeenth-century Zen master, can be like these. The various elements support each other by a system of conventions accepted by all, for no other reason than that they have always been accepted. There may be no deep roots of conviction anywhere, but that society can look very stable. It is, however, no longer creative, and it too collapses before any sudden crisis.

In somewhat the same way, an individual personality can apparently hold together firmly, because the parts support each other. But this lasts only so long as times are good. Unless roots of spiritual conviction are put down, the whole structure is brittle and hollow and falls to pieces in a storm.

The Singing Eggs

(Translated from the Japanese of a six-year-old boy)

ONE DAY, the eggs began singing.

In the hens' nests, in the shops, in the kitchens, they were singing and singing.

The people didn't like to hear the eggs singing.

They said, "We'll cook them. We'll boil them and poach them and scramble them and fry them. Then they'll stop singing."

But even when they were boiled and poached and scrambled and fried, the eggs went on singing.

The people got angry. "We'll eat them," they said. "Then they'll have to stop singing."

But even when they were eaten, the eggs went on singing from inside the people.

The people were very angry. They were bad people.

They shouted, "We'll kill them."

They got knives and tried to kill the eggs inside them. But they only killed themselves.

And all over the world, the eggs went on singing and singing.

The Pillar

A BRILLIANT young research graduate put in for an award, and did not get even an honourable mention. He had reason to suspect jealousy in the judges. When his teacher asked him about it, he blazed out against the corruption at "the top."

"But you still want to get there?" asked the teacher.

"Well, yes. I'd like my work to be recognized."

They were sitting on chairs on the verandah, and the teacher fetched a piece of rope from the garden. He put it round one of the pillars, and passed the two ends to the pupil.

"Bring that pillar near to you."

"But that's impossible."

"Try."

The pupil stood up, braced his feet on the floor, and pulled. No result. The teacher said, "People sometimes think, if I can't get to the top, perhaps I can bring the top down to me. And they criticize and condemn, to denigrate it. But that is not the right way.

"Sit down, and lift your feet off the ground a bit. Now pull on the rope again."

At the first tug, the chair began to slide across the smooth floor, and ended up beside the pillar.

The teacher took the rope, put it back, and said no more.

The scientist pondered the incident. Some years later, another piece of his work was highly praised, and now the merit of the first piece was also recognized. A friend remarked, "You know, we all thought you were remarkably calm over that first rejection; it was a real scandal."

The researcher told him about the rope and pillar, and added confidentially, "Finally I came to realize that while I braced myself on my egoism, and tried to bring the pillar of success to me as I stood, I wouldn't succeed. When I gave up 'I' and 'here,' my efforts had their natural result. The teacher did it in that special way: considering the state I was in, I don't think sermons would have had much effect."

Unseen

THERE IS a certain commercialism in some aspects of the Western world-view, extending into religion and art as well as home life and the business of making a living, where it is to be expected.

One result is that where an action done, or a mere existence, leads to no quantifiable result in human terms, it tends to be written off as entirely futile.

There is another view in the East (strongly subscribed to though not necessarily carried out in practise), in which an action rightly performed, or a true existence (as distinct from an imitation), has a sufficient value in itself. It may lose much of that value by being mixed up with ideas of results.

This view is expressed in the Gita verse:

Let your concern be with right action,
Never with getting its fruits;
Let not desire for fruits be your motive,
But do not be attached to inaction.

Some Westerners believe that without a desire for some subsequent result, an action will be done unenthusiastically or even carelessly. If results do not matter, then the cleaner will leave spots and smears on the floor; the results do not matter, so why clean well? One reply to this is that in that case the action has not in fact been done. If the floor is not clean, it has not in fact been done. If the floor is not clean, it has not been cleaned. One who has to be motivated by expectation of results, whether rewards, appreciation, or fear, is called a man of Rajas or passion-struggle, and Rajas always leads to pain in the end.

A famous expression of that pain is the gentle melancholy of Gray's verse:

Full many a gem of purest ray serene,
The dark unfathom'd caves of ocean bear:
Full many a flower is born to blush unseen,
And waste its sweetness on the desert air.

Baudelaire adapted, and perhaps enriched, the last two lines; but the idea is the same sadness and futility:

Mainte fleur épanche à regret
Son parfum doux comme un secret
Dans les solitudes profondes.

And many a rueful flower must waste
Its sweet perfume, as a secret
On deserts no man ever trod.

The whole feeling is transformed into peace by the Japanese verse on the same theme:

Not for the sake of a beholder,
In the deep mountains
Blossoms the cherry
Out of the sincerity of its heart.

www.ingramcontent.com/pod-product-compliance
Lightning Source LLC
Chambersburg PA
CBHW041257040426
42334CB00028BA/3059